Get Laid Now!
The Man's Guide to Picking Up Women and Casual Sex

Get Laid Now!
The Man's Guide to Picking Up Women and Casual Sex

By

Tab Tucker

New Tradition Books

Get Laid Now!
The Man's Guide to Picking Up Women and Casual Sex.
by
Tab Tucker

New Tradition Books
ISBN 1932420576
All rights reserved
Copyright © 2006 by Tab Tucker.
This book may not be reproduced in whole or in part without written permission.

For information contact:
New Tradition Books
newtraditionbooks@yahoo.com

Disclaimer: This book is not intended to replace medical advice or be a substitute for a psychologist. The author and publisher expressly disclaim responsibility for any adverse affects of this book. Neither author nor publisher is liable for information contained herein. It is up to the reader to take precautions against sexually transmitted diseases. Always practice safe sex.

Contents

Get Laid Now! This is how you do it. 1
You're not a eunuch. Don't act like one. 3
Setting your goals. 5
What will get you laid. 7
Picking up women is not a magical process. 11
Easy women and some of their characteristics. 14
Overcoming the Sleaze Factor 18
Proceed with caution: Safe Sex. 20
Health Screenings. A good thing. 22
You will have to stand out in the crowd. 23
Location. Location. Location. 24
Places where you *will not* get laid. 26
Confidence. 29
Great places to find easy women: Swing clubs. 32
It's the presentation that counts. 34
How to approach women 37
Pick-up lines? Are you kidding? 41
Developing your script. The art of small talk. 43
Self-control. 47
The importance of staying sober. 50
How to make her want you. 51
The best guy in the room: Your clothes. 53
The best guy in the room: Hygiene and grooming. 57
The best guy in the room: Your physical appearance. 60
Great places to find easy women: Hotel bars. 62
Don't aim too high. 64
Internet options. The easiest way to get laid? 67
Chivalry is not dead. The way to keep getting laid. 71
How to know if she's ready. 73
How to seal the deal. 75
No means no. How to handle rejection. 78
Great places to find easy women: The Club. 81

- The much celebrated, but greatly overrated wingman......... 83
- Friends with benefits?... 85
- Girls' night out? I don't think so. 87
- Do you wanna be in pictures? 89
- Dirty tricks 91
- Great places to find easy women: Nudist resorts................... 94
- Let the big head do the thinking.. 97
- Great places to find easy women: Science fiction conventions. 100
- Bad boys versus nice guys... 102
- Spring break?.. 104
- Prostitutes... 105
- The Mercy Fuck. A myth that will not get you laid. 108
- But what if she wants a real relationship?............................. 110
- What we've learned.. 111
- In conclusion.. 115

Get Laid Now! This is how you do it.

Everybody wants some!

Yes, it's true that everyone wants to get laid. The only trouble is that it's not as easy as most people would like. They go through life searching for that perfect pick-up line or that special scent (body spray, anyone?) that will get a woman into bed in the as easily as they unlock the next level of their favorite video game. But this is just wrong thinking and actually makes the act of getting laid much harder than it should be.

In a word, these people are clueless.

They don't realize that the secret of getting laid is not in finding some sort of mystic mojo that will put them through to the next level. The secret is that it's all up to them. Along with the basic knowledge of knowing where to look for *easy, available women*—a term I, in no way mean to be disrespectful—the secret mainly lies in how a person presents himself when he finds himself in the right place at the right time. You don't go to a lemon tree to pick apples, do you? You go to the apple tree, right? The same principle applies to getting laid. A friend once told me, *"If you want to get smarter, you hang around with smarter people. If you want to get laid, you hang around with sluts."* It's that simple. If you want to get some, you have to go to where the women are willing and easy. You have to go to the places where they're just as horny as you are. And you have to know what to do when you find them.

And that's what this book is going to help you do—find easy, available women. It's also going to tell you what to do to put yourself in the front of the pack of all the other guys who are there for the same reason. It will also save you a lot of time and effort by revealing to you the in's and out's of casual sex and whether or not it's even worth it to you to engage in it. Regardless, you're going to know what it's about and how to do it.

If you're looking for a serious relationship, this is not necessarily the book for you. Sure, something might develop out of one of your possible, future escapades, but that's not the purpose of this book. This book is about enabling you to get down and dirty. It's about helping you achieve that one thing that keeps eluding you in life. This book is for the guys who don't want to bother with wining and dining. What I'm going to teach you might be considered by some to be somewhat sleazy and, honestly, it is. But that's the price you have to pay when you're out to have a good time.

The great thing about what I'm going to show you is that, once you get started, your confidence will soar and when it does, you're going to get laid even more. But first we've got to get you started. I hope you're ready.

You're not a eunuch. Don't act like one.

First off, before you do anything else, you're going to have to come to terms with the fact that if you want to have a life of casual sex, you can't go around acting like you've been neutered. Like a eunuch. You're a man, right? And you want what men want and I'm not talking about beer and ribs. I'm talking about sex.

One of the biggest problems some men have when it comes to sex is the fact that they don't want to accept their biological imperative. They can't accept the fact that sex is more important than their fantasy football team or their action figure collection. While these things are good as hobbies, they should never be more important than getting laid. These types of guys don't want to come terms with the fact that they are no longer little boys. But if you want to be a guy who gets laid, you're going to have to get over these notions. Your sex-drive should always override these interests. You've spent enough time pursuing them already, haven't you? Most women will not share these types of interests. Sure it's okay to have outside interests, but you need to be more about the getting laid than you are these other more trivial pursuits.

If you're the type of guy who takes offense when someone isn't that enthused about any of your hobbies, you probably won't be able to handle it when a woman rejects you. This is something to think about. You will need to toughen up. You need to realize that you will probably get rejected until you learn the ropes and develop your confidence. This is one thing you can count on. No one is a winner right off the bat. If you want to get laid, you will have to persevere.

To get your mind straight about casual sex, you need to understand that you're a man. You have needs. As long as you respect other people's boundaries and you and your partner are of legal age, it's okay to pursue those urges. Remember you're not a eunuch. So stop acting like one.

Setting your goals.

Before you go on the prowl, you need to figure out exactly what you want to get out of getting laid.

Yeah, of course, I know that you just want to *hit it*, but there's a little more to it than that. You need to figure out if you want a relationship or just an easy lay. This book is about the easy lay. It's about the guy who doesn't have time (or doesn't want to take the time) to really get to know a girl. Sure a relationship can develop but that's another subject entirely. Also you need to figure out if you're the kind of guy who can even have casual sex. And by *casual sex* I mean no-strings attached sexual relations between consenting adults of legal age. Some people feel intense guilt over such trysts. You need to figure out if you're the kind of guy who's going to fall in love with every girl you have sex with or are going to look at it as just a good time. If you're the kind of guy who easily falls in love and becomes obsessed, casual sex is not for you. After all, you don't want to put yourself in the position where you become viewed as some kind of stalker. Remember, it's about two people having fun. You have to keep focused on the fact that you're out for the sex and that's it. There's nothing wrong with this line of thinking if you both know from the get-go that's what you're after.

All this leads to the fact that when you're looking for casual sex, it's good to know some basic rules.

Rules for Casual Sex

- It has no meaning.
- You're not looking for a relationship.
- Everybody needs to have a good time. Not just you or her.
- Don't become obsessed.
- Always use protection and practice safe sex.

These rules are very simple so there's no need to complicate them. It's just a tryst, a one-night stand, so it shouldn't have any meaning other than the sex. Casual sex has nothing to do with forming an emotional relationship and if it's not fun for everyone, why do it? That is pretty much the gist of casual sex. Keep these rules in mind at all times, and your mind will be in the right place when you're on the hunt. It's when people forget these rules that someone inevitably gets disappointed or hurt.

Another thing you need to think about is your expectations. Are you looking to bed Miss America? Or are you just looking for a piece? If you're looking for Miss America, good luck! So is every other guy out there. But if you're looking for a girl that you might actually have a shot with, then you're in luck. Setting your goals and priorities is very important when you're starting on a path of casual sex. If you aren't realistic, you'll just be wasting your time. You don't want to do that, do you?

What will get you laid.

The question of what will get a person laid has been one that has puzzled man since the beginning of time. Men wonder just what will unlock a woman's desires so that she will be willing to have sex with them. Is it something magical? Is it something psychological? Is it something physical? Is it some kind of hypnosis? Just what is it exactly?

While the answer to this question is easy, executing it is sometimes a little more difficult. As I have already briefly alluded to earlier, the thing that will get you laid is *you*. *Just you.* Sure, the location is extremely important, but what if you find yourself in the *Land of Loose Women* and you don't know what to do? You're just going to be passed over for every other guy there. This is why you have to make yourself into a guy with whom women want to have sex. However, getting you to this point is another story entirely. Some of you guys will not have much trouble with this. You will be able to take advice and constructive criticism. However, others of you will think that you're perfect already. You will think that your too-short short pants show off your great legs. Or that your *Lord of the Rings* fixation is a good conversation starter. For you people, good luck. Remember, when it comes to your clothes and conversation, you're trying to find common ground and you don't want her to classify you too early on. Most women are not really into this stuff and may consider you to be a little nerdy if you express these interests or wear unstylish clothes. You have to learn keep these self-sabotaging impulses at bay. This is why you have to recognize that you do not know everything and that sometimes it is good to listen to advice. Until you can realize that there's a reason why you're not getting laid, you're just going to be spinning your wheels.

But before we go any farther, you need to come to terms with the fact that there are three essential things about yourself that you will need to come to grips with before you start looking for casual sex.

- You have to be a guy with whom women want to have sex.
- You have to go to know where the easy women are.
- You have to know what to do when you get there.

I'm going to cover all these subjects throughout the course of this book, but as I said earlier, the one unifying element on this list is you. Yes, it's all up to you. You will play a very crucial role in getting your sex life started. Some people will insist that there's some sort of pick-up line that will magically unlock the Garden of Eden. Just say some magic words and she'll start lusting after you. Think again. There are no such words. Others will think that they can trick a woman into having sex with them, that they can put on a sob story and make a woman feel sorry for them or that they can coerce a woman into a sexual encounter. While it is possible to play on a woman's sympathy to have sex with you, I wouldn't count on it. You're treading on dangerous ground here. You will make yourself someone's bad memory and if word of your manipulation gets around, you will definitely be a marked man. You might even wind up in jail if you deceive her so badly that she looks at what you did to her as rape.

Also, there are people who think that they can simply talk a woman into having sex with them. They think that they can go about it in a similar fashion as they would if they were trying to convince her to buy a used car. I'm here to let you know that this is just a waste of time. Unless a woman is easy already (and doesn't require you to talk her into it), you will not talk her into a one night stand. If you're planning on spending a lot of time and money on her, then you might stand a chance. But why would you do that if all you want is to have sex? There are plenty of women out there who won't require all that work.

As I keep saying, the bottom line when it comes to getting laid is *you*. You will be the catalyst that makes her want to go to bed with you. Do you have to be the best looking guy out there? No, you don't. However, you will have to be well-groomed. You will have to be well-dressed and you will have to be charming. You will also have to act like you're interested in her as a person. You will also have to be a gentleman. A woman wants to have sex with a guy who's a winner and if you can put out the vibe that you are a guy that it's okay for her to have sex with, she will be more likely to have sex with you. Above all, you will have to be willing to expend the effort. Of course, as with anything, while there are no guarantees, whatever you can do to increase your chances is a good thing.

Throughout the course of this book, we'll go over various aspects of self-improvement that will assist you in your quest to be a ladies' man. But be prepared that it will require some work. Some of you will need less work than others. Some of you will require just a little tweaking and some of you will need a complete overhaul. But don't be intimidated. Everything that needs to be done to make you a ladies' man is within your reach. You just have to make the effort. Remember, I'm not trying to make you over into a guy who's looking for serious relationship. You are not trying to be *Mr. Right* or *The One*. You're just trying to be *Mr. Right Now*. I'm just going to help you to *be the man,* so to speak, for a one night stand. The women you're going to go after aren't looking for a serious relationship—period. All they want is a good time. And you have to be a guy that they can feel good about having a good time with.

How you present yourself is key in having a successful one-night stand. If you're trying to sell a house, you would take the trouble to clean and decorate it in order to get the best price, wouldn't you? So why be hesitant about taking the same pains with yourself? No one knows it all and if you can put your ego aside for just a little while as you read this book, you might just learn something that can get you laid on a regular basis.

That's not too much to ask, is it?

Picking up women is not a magical process.

When it comes to picking up women, one of the hardest things for guys to grasp is that it is not a magical process. There is not some sort of mystical incantation that you can utter (I'm talking pick-up lines here) that will make a woman want to go to bed with you. It is a process, plain and simple. It is a routine. And all it takes is work and practice and anyone can do it. There is no hocus pocus involved.

While some guys may have an easier time getting laid than others due to the fact that they're in better shape, better looking, etc., it is still a skill that anyone can master. Your level of commitment is very crucial. This is not something at which you can make a half-hearted stab and a sigh of resignation. You will have to work at it. But let me preface my comments by first saying that the better you dress, the more well-groomed and buff you are and the more confidently you present yourself, the easier it will be for you. It's just like running a marathon. The stronger you are, the more easily you'll finish. You can be weak and still finish, but it will be much more difficult and you'll probably finish last.

So, how do you acquire this skill? How do you learn how to pick up women? You start out by being yourself. That is to say, the best version of yourself you can be. This is how you develop your approach: If you're a funny guy, use humor. If you're a smart guy, use your intellect. It's all you and if you can just be yourself, you will come off as a much more confident guy. If you have a nice smile, loosen up and show those teeth. This is what the women like—confidence. Some guys think that if they pretend to be some sort of royalty or movie or sports star or something, it'll get them laid. This might work in the movies, but in the real world, most women are going to see right through it and you'll only end up looking like a fool.

You'll also have to learn to talk to women without being intimidated by them. You can't mushmouth around. It's like a job interview. You have a very short time to make a first impression and most easy women know within a few minutes whether or not you're worth sleeping with. Remember, you're not the only guy in the room so make any time you get to talk to the girl count. Convince her you're worthy without wearing her down. This doesn't mean that you have to tell her your life story. Just let her know (without actually coming out and saying it) that you're a cool, confident guy who's good to party with. If you give her too many tedious details, she'll only get bored with you. It doesn't take much, just a confident smile and knowing what and what not to say. You can do this by just being yourself. There's no need to lie about how you help feed orphans or save whale habitats. This stuff will only come back on you.

Another good skill to have is to know when to tone it down. Try to be observant enough to know if you're overpowering her in the conversation or annoying her with your presence. Don't be too oversensitive, but look for the subtle signs that she's not digging you and move on. If she is constantly inching away from you or looking at someone else or at her watch, chances are, you're wasting your time. This is when you need to give it up and move on before you embarrass yourself. Believe me, if you persist, you'll look back at this moment and cringe.

Most guys who get laid a lot are just being themselves. They're able to open up enough to let the world see who they are. Women like men who are genuine. Sure they sometimes like assholes too, but not necessarily if they have options. (See chapter on *Bad Boys versus Nice Guys.*) The thing for you to realize is that anyone can get laid. It's not something that's going to take decades of study in a Tibetan monastery. All it takes is for you to get out there in the world and go for it. Sure, you'll get shot down a few times, but look at this rejection as practice. You'll get better and better as you fine-tune your game and learn from your mistakes. After reading the book, you'll be armed with the knowledge to know what you're doing wrong and make the necessary adjustments. And if you keep knocking at the door long enough, more than likely, you'll be allowed to enter.

Easy women and some of their characteristics.

When you're getting started on your road to free and easy casual sex, it's a good thing to learn the types of women you're going to be looking for. And when it comes to casual, free sex, the types of women you will be looking for will have to be of the *easy* variety.

When I use the term *easy women*, let me point out that I, in no way, mean this to be disrespectful. Easy women are ladies and should be treated as such, with the utmost respect. They are not to be looked down upon or treated as tramps or low-class trash. They are not cheap. They just like sex and are not afraid to have it. They are the life's blood of getting laid. They are just like us in regard to their sex-drive. They just have to the power over whether or not it actually happens.

As I said before, you're not going to be going for Miss America—unless, of course, she falls into one of these categories. These are the types of women who are going to be doing it with *someone* and your goal is to be *the someone* with whom they're doing it.

Most easy women fall into several broad categories. Some more than one. You will find them everywhere. At the night club, the frat party, the swing club, anywhere you find women, in fact. They can be artsy-fartsy, hippie chicks, socialites, science nerds or the girl-next-door. The important

Easy women and some of their characteristics. 15

thing is that if you can classify, you can identify. Especially due to the fact that you can encounter these various types of women in almost any setting. Remember, while they are loose, they are still people so it makes sense that they will be in the places that people usually congregate.

Here's the main types of easy women you'll encounter:

The Exhibitionist: This is the girl who loves to take her clothes off at the party. She's always showing off her body to get attention. The biggest problem with her is that she may be a bit of a tease. She might want you to look but not touch. If this happens, don't get upset; just be glad you got to enjoy the show.

The Revenge Fucker: This is the girl who's just using you to get back at her boyfriend/husband. This type of girl is especially good if you don't want a relationship. Don't feel bad if she's not that into it or makes you fell like a piece of meat. This is what you are to her. Be glad she found you. Also watch out for her significant other. He might be the jealous type.

The Swinger: Of course, you know this type. She can also fall into the same category as the *Exhibitionist*. This girl is the wife/girlfriend who is being swapped. She knows what she wants and you need to be the guy to give it to her. She wants casual sex. She wants group sex. She wants any kind of sex. She's a good, easy lay; just don't be surprised if her husband/boyfriend wants to watch. Also see *Hotwife*.

The Hotwife: This one is similar to the *Swing*er, but most likely is playing some sort of game with her husband where she goes out and screws strange men and then goes back and tells him about it. If you can find one of these, you're in like Flynn, but if you can't handle the sleaze factor, you might want to skip her.

The Thrill Seeker: This is the type of woman you're likely meet at the hotel bar. She's probably married or in a relationship but wants something more on the side. If you can avoid feeling used, you'll be fine.

The Rebel: Similar to the *Thrill Seeker*, but is usually younger. This is the girl who's rebelling against her daddy by having sex with everything and anything that moves. She usually comes from a religious background. She's a good time, but try not to question why having sex with you is something she considers radical.

The Nympho: This is the girl with problems. She just can't get enough sex. She's got a huge hole she's trying to fill and no number of men will be able to fill it. She's probably got a lot of issues and will want to have sex within a short time of meeting you. She does it because she wants you to like her and she thinks the only thing she has to offer is sex. She's an easy way to go, if you can handle the weight of her low self-esteem. If you do decide to go for it, I hope you don't mind company. You may have to take your turn.

Most easy women fall into at least one of these categories. Sometimes they can fall into several. Of course, there are some subgroups which I haven't listed, but these pretty much cover it. I've chosen not to include categories like *Unhappily Married Women* and *Wallflowers* because they will require more work than you want to put out. This book is not about seduction. It's about *getting laid*.

Since you now know the categories, you'll be more likely to detect when you're in the presence of an easy woman. You can encounter them in any setting, so it's that much more important to recognize them when you see them. You might even want to go to bars, parties, swing clubs, etc. and observe these types of women in action in order to become more accustomed to what they are about. Your route to casual sex will be all the easier if you do your homework. Studying doesn't have to be boring. (At least not when it comes to observing human behavior.) Knowledge is power, especially if it's going to help get you laid.

Overcoming the Sleaze Factor.

Let's face it. Casual sex can be kind of sleazy. You're hooking up with strangers—or people who are almost strangers—for the sole purpose of unencumbered sex and nothing else. You're following your lower impulses and probably abandoning a good portion of your upbringing. It can make you feel a little cheap and used if you let it.

If you have a problem with guilt over sexual matters or have a strong moral compass, casual sex is probably not your thing. Sure, you may fantasize about it, but the reality of the situation will probably be a lot less spectacular and much dirtier than your fantasy. Know yourself. If you're the type of person who has a hard time watching porn, then casual sex is not for you.

But what if you don't have these issues? What if you're a free spirit? If this is the case, how can you overcome the *Sleaze Factor?* It's simple as far as casual sex goes, you just need to look at the benefits versus the costs.

Look at it this way: You're taking a risk of feeling cheap and used, but you are able to get your rocks off and achieve that feeling of sexual conquest. You're taking a chance on catching a disease (always wear a condom and practice safe sex!) but you might be able to bed that hot chick you've been drooling over. You're running the risk of your friends and family thinking you're a slimeball, but you're getting laid on a regular basis. I think you get my point here.

Everything has a price and the price of casual sex may be feeling like a sleaze. Remember to know yourself and compensate accordingly. If you feel cheap, empower yourself that you were able to hit that thing. If you're worried about people thinking badly of you, be discreet and don't talk about your numerous sexual exploits. Most of your trepidations can be overcome if you can just think of a way to justify them.

Overcoming the *Sleaze Factor* is very achievable. You just have to be self-aware enough to know your limitations and guard accordingly. Just don't do anything you're going to hate yourself in the morning for and you'll be all right.

Proceed with caution: Safe Sex.

When you're embarking upon a life of casual sex, the number one thing you need to do is protect yourself. If you're not the kind of guy who likes to wear a condom then you're not the kind of guy who needs to go around having casual sex.

It's that simple.

I know that it feels better when a condom is not involved, but the risks are just too great. Sex with strangers can be risky and no woman, no matter how hot or how easy, is worth risking your health. It doesn't matter if she says it's okay for you not to wear one. The thing to remember is if she says it's okay not to wear one when she's with you, she's probably also saying it with every other guy she's sleeping with.

Wearing a condom and practicing safe sex are crucial if you're going to be promiscuous. Most women will be glad that you insist on wearing a condom and if they insist you don't, you might want to think twice about having sex with them. There are some women who will say that it's okay for you not to wear a condom just so long as you get an HIV test. I wouldn't buy this if I were you. Remember that she's probably telling this to every other guy she's screwing. You need to realize that HIV tests can sometimes be wrong. Also, HIV can't even be tested for until several months after a person is infected. In other words, there's a window where a person can have it without it showing up on a test. All it takes is for one person in such a situation to have sex with you or the person with whom you're going to have sex for you to potentially contract HIV. It's just not worth it. Wear the condom. If you're unsure of the particulars of proper condom use and safe sex practices, consult your local health department or personal physician.

Another reason you want to protect yourself is that you do not want to get a girl pregnant under these conditions. It's not worth the increased sensation to put yourself in a situation where you're going to have to make decisions that can radically influence the rest of your life or mental well-being.

If, somehow, your casual tryst develops into a serious relationship, the condom situation should probably come up for discussion between the two of you. However, make sure that you both have health screenings and fully understand that having sex without a condom means a higher level of commitment in the relationship. If you're not ready for this, keep wearing one.

So before you stick it in, put on a condom. It's the smart thing for you to do. If she insists otherwise, I would think twice about her. You wouldn't play catch without a baseball glove would you? So why should you have sex with a stranger without a condom?

Health Screenings. A good thing.

I've already gone over why you need to wear a condom whenever you have sex. Even so, it's a good idea to have a routine health screening if you manage to develop a lifestyle of casual sex. It's just the smart thing to do. You need to get checked for the various venereal diseases along with HIV. It's better to know and get treated than it is to live in ignorance and let conditions worsen.

Athletes get routine check ups. So why shouldn't a person who engages in casual sex? There's nothing to be afraid of, it's just part of the game. If you want to play, you have to be ready. Health screenings insure that you're always doing the right thing by yourself and the partner with whom you choose to have sex.

You will have to stand out in the crowd.

One very important thing to remember when you're only out to get laid is that there will be far more men who are just looking for casual sex than there are women. Regardless of the Sexual Revolution, the amount of horny guys is always going to be greater than the number of horny girls. Whether you go to the club or are looking to hook up via the internet, you are always going to be just one of many. But you need to realize that while this can be daunting, you can also use it to your advantage. Make use of the fact that so many of these other horny guys are absolutely clueless as to how to get laid. Many of them think all they have to do is show up. You will know differently after reading this book. You will know what easy women are looking for and how to satisfy those needs. Being one of many is only a disadvantage if you allow yourself to remain in the *many* category. Be the one. This is your goal. You have to be the diamond in the rough, so to speak.

So be aware that the pickings can be a little slim when it comes to casual sex. But don't despair. There are plenty of women out there who are looking for the same thing as you. This is why you have to make yourself stand out. If you can do this, picking up easy, good-time seeking women out from under the noses of all the losers out there will be like taking candy from a baby.

Location. Location. Location.

If you're looking for fish, you don't go to the desert, do you? Well, the same philosophy applies to getting laid. If you're not looking in the right places, you're just going to be spinning your wheels.

One of the biggest problems with many of these types of books that attempt to tell you how to get laid is that they simply aren't realistic. They confuse the notion of meeting women with the much more focused idea of *meeting women who want to get laid.*

What I mean by this is, you can meet a girl at the park or grocery story and then have a nice conversation or maybe a date afterwards but it doesn't necessarily mean that she's going to put out. Sure, some women in some of these places are going to want to get it on, but the percentage is very small. In fact, it's about like hitting the lottery. This is because the context is all wrong. She's at the grocery store to buy something to eat, not hook up and have crazy sex with some guy she's just met.

But where does a fellow go to meet these kinds of women?

That's what I'm going to tell you through the course of this book. There are places that are guaranteed to have a higher percentage of horny women. Are all women in these places open for business? No, but many of them will be. And that's all you need to know. Anything that can increase the likelihood of you getting laid is definitely a good thing.

Easy women don't grow on trees. That's why you don't look for them there. Location is probably one of the most important elements when it comes to getting laid. If you don't go to where the easy women are, it's going to be that much harder for you to embark on your lifestyle of casual sex.

Places where you *will not* get laid.

As I've mentioned before, location is probably one of the biggest factors in your quest for casual sex. If you don't go where the easy women are, you're just wasting your time and energy on something that is not going to happen. While we'll get into some of the places where you're most likely to find easy women later in the book, I think it's also important to explore the places where you're most likely *not to get laid*.

Yes, it's true. There are some places where, because of false information put out by numerous teen exploitation movies and porno movies, you would think that you would have an easy time of it. However, you would be wrong. While, of course, there are the typical ones, like churches or the hardware store—I'm not going to go into these—there are others that would *seem* to have easy women galore. But, alas, no. This is just not the case.

Places where you will not get laid:
Strip clubs: This one should be a no-brainer, but many guys go into these establishments with the idea that the strippers will fall in love with them. Or that, because these girls take their clothes off, they will be easy lays. Allow me to let you in a cold hard fact. Unless the girl is earning something on the side by prostituting herself, most likely, she'll only talk to you until your money runs out. Most strippers have absolutely no respect for the men who come into strip clubs. They look at them as guys who aren't capable of being able

to look at naked women any other way. So, when you go to a strip club, just go with the intention of looking at some naked women. These girls are there to earn their living. Besides, most of them are already in some sort of relationship with someone else. Don't think she's digging you just because she sits and talks to you all night. She's only after what's in your wallet. Besides, many strippers prefer women sexually. A lot of them don't even like men. And don't even think about trying anything funny with one of the girls, otherwise the bouncers will gladly show you the way out—the hard way, on your ass.

That place that serves hot-wings where the girls wear orange shorts: Ah, *that place that serves hot-wings where the girls wear orange shorts* is, in my opinion, the home of sub-par food and crappy service. If you've ever been into one of these places at all, you've probably noticed how the waitresses seem to absolutely detest you. Well, there's a reason for this. They do. All they're after is the tip. They figure if they're going to be objectified by wearing those skimpy outfits, they don't have to be nice. Just look at the place as merely a bar with scantily clad waitresses and bad service. Because essentially that's what it is. Don't overtip and you'll be okay. Remember, these chicks are working there to earn a living not to take you home. (This information applies to those bars where the waitresses act *crazy*, insult you and get up and dance on top of the bar as well.)

The Grocery Store: I think the myth of the grocery story hook-up started on some sit-com in the mid-seventies. Ever since then, you always see the grocery store brought up as a great place to meet women. To the perpetuators of this myth: Have you ever actually been to a grocery store? Most of the time the only women there are moms and grandmas. Go for the groceries, not the casual sex.

The Nude Beach: While it would make sense that the nude beach would be a great place to pick up loose women, this would probably be true if women actually *went* to the nude beach. If you ever get over your initial fears of being nude in public and take that plunge, you'll unfortunately find that most of the people at the nude beach are men. Any women who are there are most likely with their husbands or boyfriends. And while some of these women will be open for business, this will probably be such a rare occasion that you would have had better luck if you had gone to a regular beach. If you go to the nude beach, just enjoy the sand and sun. Just hope to see a few nude women and try to ignore all the dudes there. (Please bear in mind that not all nudist-oriented places are bad places to look for casual sex. See the chapter on *Nudist resorts* for more information.)

While there are more places where you can pretty much guarantee that you won't get laid, I just wanted to hit the high spots to give you examples of what I'm talking about. The main thing to recognize is that location is just as important in knowing where not to look for easy women as it is in looking for easy women. It's better to learn from other people's mistakes. So believe me when I say, if you can avoid the spots where you *will definitely not* get laid, you will definitely increase your chances of having casual sex

Confidence.

Regardless of what you're going for in life, confidence is a quality that can absolutely help facilitate what you're trying to achieve. Whether your goal is in business, sports or your interactions with others, it can really make a difference. This is true of normal dating, but it's especially true of dating for casual sex.

Women love men who are sure of themselves and know what they want. They like men who are comfortable with who they are and who are not afraid to take charge. If you can be confident when you meet a woman with whom you want to have sex, it shows. And the object of your desires is going to notice.

It's a fact that men have to be confident in order to get laid regularly. What's weird is that this is not the case for women. The truth of the matter is that a lot of women have sex because they're insecure while an insecure man will hardly, if ever, get laid. It's just not fair, is it? But that's just the way it is. One thing to remember, though, is that you can't confuse confidence with cockiness or conceit. Confidence doesn't mean that you have to think that you're God's gift to women, but having a quiet assurance in yourself. It's knowing that you belong and that you know what to do in the situation. It's about handling yourself like you're ready for anything the world presents to you. It's a delicate balance to achieve, but it is possible.

You may have been told that it's great to act all bashful and *"aw-gee-shucks"* in order to tempt women into trying to seduce you. This is not good advice. While it might work once in a blue moon, most likely she'll just go off with the confident, self-assured guy. You're trying to do things that are more likely to get you laid, remember? This is why you have to raise the likelihood that you will get laid. Doing things that are hit and miss will only lower your chances. Always go for the sure thing. And by acting confident, you will definitely up your odds.

So how do you get confidence? You've heard the old phase, *"Fake it until you make it?"* Well, that's pretty much it. If you don't have it, act like you have it because if you act long enough, you will have it. It's that simple. You just have to develop the habit of being confident. Role play if you have to. Find a role model and emulate him. Pretend you belong wherever you go. Pretend you can kick every man's ass in the place. Pretend that you've got an extremely large penis. Anything that makes you feel like a bad ass. Of course, you can't go around saying this stuff aloud. Just pretend to yourself and adopt that quiet confidence you need to get laid. Keep in mind that women *expect* a man to be confident. It's up to you to actually be confident. Acting like you belong in a place is the key. If you can do this and get to the point where you're getting laid regularly, your confidence will soar. You will quickly form new habits and pretty soon your role playing and pretending will become second nature. It's all about getting into a new groove. You need to remember that this woman is getting something from you, too. She's probably pretty insecure herself, so don't think of her as being anything better than you. Everybody has the capacity to be confident, they just have to push through the pain, so to speak, and get to it.

And what if you're already a confident person? Just count your lucky stars and go with the flow. Just try not to come off as being arrogant. Women love confident men, but they hate conceited jerks. They just love to put men like this in their place and do so at every opportunity.

Remember, confidence is the foundation on which your promiscuous future lies. Develop it and it will definitely get you laid.

Great places to find easy women: Swing clubs.

I'm sure you know all about those people referred to as *swingers*. I'm not talking about dancing, either. They're the married/committed couples who get off on swapping sexual partners. It's also called wife-swapping and it's a great way for a guy to get laid without much effort. And even better than this, these people have clubs where they go to *swing* and *swap* and have lots of casual sex.

But if it's called *wife-swapping*, how's a single guy supposed to get in on the action?

It's easy. You go to the swing clubs on *single-guy* night. Yes, you heard me. Single-guy night. While many swinging couples detest the idea of single men because they're generally pushy and don't know when to take no for an answer, there are some couples who don't mind single men. In fact, they seek them out. These women are sometimes into group sex or they're just looking for a third. Your job is to tread lightly, be nice to everyone, treat everyone with respect and let the couples who are interested come to you.

It's really that simple.

But the downside of it is, as I mentioned earlier, is that many couples are suspicious of single guys. A few bad apples have ruined the whole bunch due to the fact that many of them, when they go to swing clubs, act like the women are there only to have sex with them. This is not the case. As with anything, the woman has to be attracted to you. (See the chapter, *It's the presentation that counts*.) The same rules apply as in any casual sex situation. If you want to get laid, you have to be a guy with whom a woman wants to have sex. This leads to another one of the drawbacks of swing clubs on single-guy night. There will be many more guys there than couples or women. This is even more reason to make sure that you are the best that you can be. Because, believe me, most of the guys there won't have a clue.

As far as finding swing clubs, you'll have to look places other than your local yellow pages. These establishments are fairly low-key. However, if you go to websites that are geared towards swingers, you can usually search for the swing clubs in your area or you can find the resources which will help you do so. You can also find out lots of information on swinging etiquette and terminology from these sites. Remember swingers are very social and want as many people as they can to join in. But be aware, these places are not cheap. Especially for single guys. You will have to pay for the pleasure of attending a place where the sex comes this easily.

In the swing club, the biggest thing to remember is to be polite. Always treat the couples with respect. Especially the women. If a woman is interested in you, she'll let you know. Remember, she's in control. You're the one who is on display. If you can be a nice, polite guy who has it together as far as his style of dress and hygiene and manners go, you'll stand a very good chance of getting laid, or at least a blowjob.

So, if you want an easy way to get laid, try a swing club. Just be aware that, in order to get laid, you may have to participate in some sort of group sex situation. Maybe not, but if you're game for something like this, go for it. Just be sure to wear a condom. And always be a gentleman.

It's the presentation that counts.

Think about it. How often do you judge people by how they look? Before you even get the chance to talk to them? How many times do you assess them as being losers? As dumbasses? As jerks? And you do this over the course of just a few minutes or even seconds in some cases. Well, this should tell you something about first impressions. If you're going to get laid, you have to make a good first impression.

Now, I know that many of you guys have had mothers who have taught you that a girl should love you for who you are on the inside. That it's all about your personality and your wit and your soul. Well, this may technically be the ideal situation, but when it comes to casual sex, it's all about presentation and the outside appearance. If you don't come off as a guy who's ready for a good time and is able to give a good time, you're going to be spending a lot of time with yourself. If you don't want to accept this fact, you're only going to grow more and more frustrated as the years tick by. While loving someone for who they are on the inside is a very warm, fuzzy, romantic way of looking at things, it is very unrealistic when it comes to casual sex. You also need to know that this comes from romance novels and chick flicks.

Everyone knows that first impressions are important when it comes to business, so why is getting laid any different? How can a woman even begin to fathom sleeping with you if she hates the way you dress? A person who takes this *come-as-you-are* approach is asking a lot without giving much in return. This is just a lazy way to approach picking up women and lazy never gets laid.

So, how do you make a good first impression? It's easy. Try to look and act your best. Forget your favorite football jersey and go with a nice shirt. Try not to dress like a little boy. Forget the sneakers and wear adult shoes. Dress like a guy who knows what's going on at the club. Women love clothes and they particularly appreciate a guy who knows how to dress. We'll discuss the particulars of this in a later chapter.

Also, have a good introduction lined up. Don't be awkward and unprepared. If you don't have something to say, you'll just stumble and stammer. This may make you look sweet and shy (if you're lucky) but don't count on it. Remember, the mercy fuck is a myth. (See chapter on *The Mercy Fuck*.) You need to look like a guy who's in control. Don't be too afraid to spend a buck. Buy the girl a drink. Easy women usually love to drink and alcohol loosens them up even more. They want to party. Be ready to bring it.

And, of course, always try to be a gentleman. Ask any woman. Most guys are jerks. They all come off as just wanting to screw a girl and if she isn't willing to jump into the sack at the mere sight of them, they get pissed off. Set yourself apart. Open her door. Buy her a drink. Compliment her clothing. While you are looking to get laid, you'll be much more successful if you act like you're also interested in her as a person. This is fine line, though. Don't overdo it. If you do, you'll be relegated to being the *friendly guy*. This is a classification that will not get you laid.

Yes, indeed, it's the presentation that counts. A good first impression is crucial for the man who seeks casual sex. All it takes is a little forethought and attention to detail to achieve that initial good impression. The thing to keep in mind is that it takes far less effort to make a good first impression than it does to try to recover from a bad one.

How to approach women.

For some men, approaching women is one of the hardest things they will ever have to do. They just don't know how to go about it. *"What am I supposed to say? How am I supposed to act? What about pick-up lines?"* These are just a few of the questions that many men have when it comes to talking to women. I understand completely, but men, if you want to get laid, you're going to have to learn how to approach women.

Here's how you do it.

The most important thing to understand is that women are people just like you. How do you like to be approached in social situations? You know what to do when you meet a co-worker, don't you? You just need to apply these same principles to the opposite sex.

You ask, *"But how do you overcome the awkwardness when it comes to meeting someone?"* This is simple. The thing to remember when it comes to approaching women, especially in a bar or other social setting, is that they're there for the same reason you are—to meet people and have fun. And better than that, easy women are there to meet people and have sex. If you can let this sink in, it will remove a lot of the awkwardness you have when it comes to approaching a complete stranger.

"But what do you say to a woman? Don't you have to know some sort of special pick-up line?" While a lot of guys

use pick-up lines, I do not recommend them. Most women, even the easiest lays in the world, will find them completely cheesy. Some guys can make them work, but it's still an extremely risky venture. The first thing you need to do is make eye contact with the object of your affection. If she looks away immediately and doesn't look in your direction again, try your luck elsewhere. However, if she looks back or quickly looks away and then gives you the look again, your chances are good. Next give her a smile. I'm not talking about a big cheesy grin either, just a little smile that tells her that you have connected with her. If she smiles back, all you need to do is go over and talk to her. This is the point that all guys dread, but speaking to a woman isn't all that difficult. All you need to say as an ice breaker is a simple, *"Hello"* or *"Hi"* or any variation of that. Just be confident when you do it, like you talk to women all the time. Like it's a given that she's going to respond favorably. Remember, you have a lot to offer and she should be glad that you're talking to her in the first place. After she says *"Hi"* back, introduce yourself and ask her if she wants a drink or, if the setting is appropriate, she wants to dance. If you're terrible dancer, wait for her to ask and then apologize for your dancing ability as you're headed to the dance floor. It'll be okay. Most women know that guys can't dance. But if you pretend to be Fred Astaire and can't back it up, you'll just look bad. So be honest. Don't ever pretend to be something you're not. (When it comes to dancing, if you want to go the extra mile and take lessons, you'll impress any woman with whom you dance.) Regardless, just go with the situation. It's this simple. If she's interested in you, she'll respond in kind and the conversation will flow. If not, it won't and you should move on to the next one.

    This leads to the next thing you need to bear in mind. If it ain't working after you offer her a drink or a dance, it ain't going to work. Period. Know when to leave the situation. If she's not responding to you in a favorable way after you start talking to her, be self-aware enough to know it. If she doesn't tell you her name after you introduce yourself or take you up on your offer of a drink or a dance, cut your losses. Be a gentleman and say that it was nice to meet her and go on to the next girl. This is probably one of the biggest problems men have when it comes to women. They simply do not know when they are not wanted. They are either self-deluded and think that they can break down a girl's defenses by relentlessly hitting on her, or they just can't get it through their thick skulls that not every woman wants them. If a girl obviously doesn't like you when you introduce yourself, she probably isn't going to like you at any point later on. In fact, it's better that you pick up the signal right away so you don't waste any more time on her. Remember that there's a lot more women out there and many of them *will be* interested in you. It's not like there's only one woman out there and you have to make her like you. Don't make every woman you meet into a conquest. Just be a gentleman if you're rejected. This girl may have friends who just might be interested in you. Always try to create a good impression with everyone and these seeds may just grow into some casual sex for you.

Casual sex will happen when you make a favorable impression with the right woman. If you cast a wide enough net, you'll get laid. You just have to remember that approaching women is a very simple thing. It's not a mystery. Just say hello with confidence and introduce yourself. If you're clicking with a girl (or she's exceptionally easy) you'll know it. And if you're wasting your time, you'll know that too. Just be self-aware enough to know the difference. These basic principles are the building blocks of getting laid. If you can't say hello to a woman, then how the hell will you be able to have sex with her? You have to start somewhere and a simple greeting is the best approach.

So when it comes to approaching women, just keep it simple. If you don't, you're taking a risk in either looking cheesy, stupid or arrogant. Remember women are people too and easy women are looking for the same thing you are. If you can just get over that initial awkwardness when it comes to meeting them, you're half-way there.

Pick-up lines? Are you kidding?

While I briefly addressed this subject previously, I thought it still deserved its own chapter. This is because it's so crucial that you completely understand how important it is for you not to use a pick-up line when you're trying to talk to a woman. Yes, when it comes to getting shot down fast, a pick-up line is a guaranteed way of making sure that you will not get laid.

Yes, you heard me. Pick-up lines will not get laid. Drill this into your head and make it a fact of life. Once you can overcome this little falsehood, you're on your way to a more fulfilling—and easier—sex life.

Here's why: Pickup lines are cheesy and generally just make you come off as looking stupid. Sure, you'll hear stories occasionally about how some guy used some really cheesy pick-up line on some girl and she was so amused that she went out with him. Yes, this does happen; however, it's extremely rare. In order to make a pick-up line work, you have to be blessed with great looks, a good body and most importantly a whole lot of confidence. Sure, a sense of humor is good too, but if that's all you've got, it's going to be an uphill struggle. Most women who are looking to get laid are not on the prowl for a man with a killer sense of timing.

It's okay to have a script somewhat rehearsed when you're talking to a girl, but you need to think of this as merely a list of talking points. Not pick-up lines. Your script should just be a list of subjects to talk about, not some silly little thing that's just going to insult her intelligence. You may have to vary it from woman to woman because not all of them will want to talk about the same thing. The thing to realize is that learning to talk to women will improve your chances and will definitely improve your chances of picking them up. You just have to be genuine. Most women can smell a rat quicker than you can drop a stupid pick-up line.

So, when it comes to pick-up lines, just a simple greeting will suffice. If you're in doubt about what I'm saying, just think about what a source of humor these things are. They have been lampooned in movies, by comedians and most importantly by the women they're used on. When you think of them in this light, they don't seem like such a good idea, do they?

Developing your script. The art of small talk.

If you're even the slightest bit shy or you are not the most confident guy in the world, it is crucial that you develop a script to follow when you're talking to women.

The script is not a litany of pick-up lines but rather a rehearsed, or semi-rehearsed, list of talking points and topics of conversation that will make it easier for you interact with new people. In other words, it's organized small-talk. Many sales people and TV talk show hosts have loose scripts developed that make the talk go much more smoothly than it would if they were just talking off the top of their heads. A good script should allow the person you're interacting with to talk about herself, which, in turn, allows you the opportunity to let the conversation flow and grow on its own accord. This allows you to relax from your script or abandon it entirely. It's done its job. It's got the ball rolling. It's also important to note (although I shouldn't have to tell you this) that a script is not something that you recite from memory like your social security number. It's very loose and just gives you an idea of something to say. It's merely a tool to get the conversation flowing. And it should be varied as needed from woman to woman. Everyone is different so you will have to adjust.

It's also very important that you don't talk too much about yourself. This will make you seem like you're self-absorbed. This can be considered a real turn-off by most women. Just keep in mind that that she's the only one who's allowed to be self-absorbed and you'll be alright. You're probably wondering why this is and think that it isn't fair that she should get to talk about herself, but you shouldn't waste time on trying to figure out why this is. Sure, it's not fair, but this is just the way it is. Look at it this way: You already know about yourself, and you want to get know her better, right? Does it not make sense to just let her talk? Of course it does. When you look at it like this, it doesn't seem quite so out of balance does it?

Of course, in your script, you must start off with a *"Hi"* or *"Hello"* or any other form of greeting. You should also smile and introduce yourself. After the greeting is when you should get into the meat of your script.

Some good things to include in your script.
- Ask her about her job.
- Compliment her on her outfit.
- Ask her where she's from.
- Ask her if she would like something to drink, eat etc.
- Ask her what's she's drinking.
- Ask her where she went to school. (This can mean high school or college, depending on the setting.)

Of course these are just suggestions and can be improved upon. You get the gist. Just keep things general and if the object of your affections is interested, these topics will spill over into much more specific conversations which will be much easier to navigate. You can respond to what she says and the conversation will take off on its own. Just keep in mind that it's all about her at first. If you can stay focused on this, you won't stumble over your words so much that it becomes awkward.

Some things not to bring up (unless she does, of course.)

- Her kids. (This might make you sound judgmental and her feel guilty about going out for casual sex.)
- If she comes to the place often. (This is a cheesy pick-up line.)
- Her family.
- If she's ever been married.
- Her ex-husband.
- If she's ever been to jail.
- Who she voted for in the last presidential election. (Or anything to do with politics. Keep in mind that if you don't share the same political views with the other person, it can be a big turn-off and even start an argument. You want casual sex, not heated bickering.)
- Where she goes to church. (Again, the guilt.)
- Sex. (This may make things so awkward that you'll never recover. You may even run her off by seeming too eager or creepy. If she wants to talk about it, let her bring it up otherwise you'll create a bad impression.)

As I mentioned earlier, it's very important for you know when a person is not receptive to you or your conversation. If she's not, don't linger. Say it was nice to meet her and move on. You'll only look bad if you stay around trying to talk to a woman who is not interested in you. There are plenty of other women who will talk to you so don't waste your time on the ones who won't.

The best way to build a script is to just pay attention when you're talking to other people, especially ones that are talkative. How do they start conversations? How does the dialogue flow? The only difference in talking to someone on the job and talking to someone in the club is that you're trying to have sex with the person at the club—unless you work in a really swinging place, of course. You can also practice by starting up conversations with people you don't know at work and other public places. After you get the hang of making small talk, it'll become that much easier to talk to women.

Remember your script is just an organized way of conducting small talk. It's that simple. If you can get an idea what you're going to say ahead of time, it will be much easier to talk to women and, hence, much easier to get laid. Small talk can lead to big things. Especially if you're trying to get laid.

Self-control.

If you're going to go out looking for casual sex, you can't view women as an all-you-can-eat buffet. You can't look at easy women with the idea that you can simply go in, hit on every single one of them and gorge yourself on their charms. It just doesn't work like this. You have to learn self-control. You have to play it cool and above all, you *can not* appear too eager. This will take a lot of self-discipline, at least in the beginning. However, once you develop this habit, it'll become second nature soon enough.

One of the main things that keep men from getting laid—especially around women who will sleep with anyone—is their eagerness. This type of man, when confronted with easy women, goes in like a dive-bomber and literally attacks the woman with propositions and attention until she is ready to run for the door. Over-eagerness is a turn-off. You must learn the fine line between eagerness and interest. You can show interest without being too eager. If you can do this, you will be much more likely to get laid.

The main way to achieve this balance is to know that your eagerness will come off as you being only interested in what *you* want. Most easy women are well aware that men want them for their bodies and not for their brains. This is why your eagerness is a turn-off for them. They know you just want to get laid. So does every other guy they meet.

What you need to do is to show interest. You do this by being interested in *her—not just yourself.* You let her talk. You ask her about her life and what she's interested in. Sure, she probably knows that you want to have sex with her, but at least you're not being a jackass. You're actually letting her talk about herself. This will allow her to let her guard down and see that you're not such a bad guy after all. This is where your self-control comes in. You have to control yourself and your desires to the point where you can suppress all that eagerness and horniness enough to allow the rational part of your brain to rule.

In order for you to develop this self-control, you will have to form new routines regarding your interaction with the opposite sex. As I mentioned earlier, a good way to do this is to develop a script to follow when speaking to a girl with whom you want to have sex. Of course, as I also mentioned earlier in the book, this isn't something you take along with you and read. This is just a list of talking points that you can bring up that will allow a woman to talk about herself. I keep reiterating this because it's just that important. Just make a mental note of other conversations you have with people you meet with whom you don't necessarily want to have sex. Then adjust for the situation. If you make a good impression, an easy woman will lead the way to casual sex. For example, you can compliment her on her outfit. Next, you can ask her about where she works, etc. It's this simple. You can modify for location or situation. If it's in a swing club, you can talk about how hot her outfit is. If it's in a bar or club, you can ask her what's she's drinking. If a person is remotely interested in you, the conversation will flow fairly naturally. Just because you want to have sex with someone doesn't mean you shouldn't be able to have a normal conversation with them as well.

Self-control. 49

Self-control is a very important of casual sex. You have to control your eagerness because no woman likes a horn-dog who is so interested in getting laid that he can't be bothered to say he likes her outfit or ask her about her work. Stay loose and don't wear your emotions on your sleeve. Just develop a list of things to talk about and you'll be fine. Once you do it enough, it'll become second-nature and you'll never be at a loss for words.

The importance of staying sober.

In any casual sex situation, it's always important to stay sober if you want to maximize your potential for getting laid. Sure, alcohol may relax you, but no woman likes a drunk. Also, when you're drunk, you're more likely to make a jackass out of yourself. Even if you're the most controlled of drinkers, there will be occasions when you will not be able to keep from making a fool out of yourself. This is okay when you're out with the guys, but remember, when it's time for casual sex, you need to stay on your game. When you're drunk and trying to get laid, you'll become pushy and you'll also miss many of the subtle opportunities to get laid that may be presented to you.

Remember you're not there for the drinking, you're there for the casual sex. You need to remember that when you're tempted to get smashed.

How to make her want you.

The good thing about picking up easy women is that they're not going to be that difficult to get into bed. That is, if they want you.

So how do you make them want you?

No matter what the setting, whether it's a date, a club, a bar, a swing club, or a nudist resort, you make them want you by being yourself or rather the *best yourself you can be*. You shouldn't act fake or like you're something you're not. You should act like a guy who's ready to have a good time. This doesn't mean to act pushy and like you're there just for one thing—sex. This kind of behavior is sure to ensure that you will not be getting any. To act like you're ready to have a good time means that you should act like you're enjoying yourself in the setting you're in. You're up for anything, but you aren't expecting anything, either. You're confident. You could take it or leave it as far as the women are concerned because you're a cool guy who's just having a good time. Women love this. It means that you are a part of the party instead of outsider-wannabe who is just trying to fit in.

You also need to talk to a woman like she's a person and not your future conquest. Just keep it light. Since women love to talk about themselves, just open up with a few general questions like *"Where are you from?"* or *"What do you do for a living?"* and she'll probably lead the conversation. (See the chapter on *Developing your script* for details.)

Women love confident men and a man who can just kick back, relax and be himself in a social situation will seem all the more confident. I'm not saying to be aloof because you will need to mingle. Just don't ever seem desperate. If you're in the presence of an easy woman, she'll let you know after you talk to her a bit. A woman who's been around the block a few times isn't going to pussyfoot around when she's feeling it and wanting to get some. Remember these aren't virgins you're with. Just relax and go with the flow.

When you combine just being loose and being yourself with a good wardrobe and good hygiene, your chances of getting laid will skyrocket. The biggest problem most men have with women is that they try to get some kind of *get laid quick scheme* going. This might work for some unscrupulous people, but most guys are just too honest to pull this kind of thing off. Remember the best *game* you have is to just be yourself. Just keep it loose and avoid any hint of desperation and you'll do great.

The best guy in the room: Your clothes.

One thing you will find out as you progress in your pursuit of casual sex is that life is not a romantic comedy and it is definitely not a porno movie. You will not just fall into sex. You will have to work at it. If it is your intention to get laid regularly, you have to turn yourself into the type of guy who gets laid regularly. This means that you have to be the best guy in the room. When you're hanging out with sluts, you have to be the guy who's good to have sex with. You have to be *the man*.

"But how do you be the man? You're not expecting me to change are you?" I'm sure that these are the thoughts that are running through your head, right?

To answer the second question first. Let's be honest, if you're reading this book, you're probably not getting laid as much as you would wish. And if this is the case, of course you're going to have to make some changes. Does that mean an extreme makeover? No, it just means fine-tuning yourself. It means that you need to tweak your image a bit in order to be the best guy in the room. In the animal kingdom, the male that stands out the most gets the mate. Think of the peacock if you have trouble visualizing this. This, of course, leads to the first question: *"How do you be the man?"* As a famous wrestler once said, *"To be the man, you have to beat the man."* And this is very much the truth. If you want to be the man who the easy women turn to for sex, you have to be, if not the best presented guy, one of the best presented guys in the room. This starts with your appearance. How you dress will play a very crucial role in your sex life.

And, yes, you may have to buy some new clothes.

But relax, this won't break you. You just need a couple of good casual outfits to wear when you go out. You can mix and match and add and subtract according to the season and occasion. The key is to keep it simple. You don't want to wear anything loud or tacky. You want your personality to be the most prominent thing about you, not your clothes. To start off, you'll need a couple of nice shirts. They can be sweaters, pull-overs or oxford cloth button-downs. Anything classic. Avoid shirts with your sports heroes and favorite teams on them. I know in the movies these shirts will lead to a fabulous relationship with some like-minded female, but you need to realize that this only happens in the movies. Most women don't like sports that much (most of them just pretend) and think men who wear these shirts when they go out are only a half-step away from being a little boy who still sleeps on his superhero sheets. You can wear them at home or when you're doing something else. Just wear a nice shirt when you go out.

As far as your pants go, go with the basics once again. Wear khakis or a dark pair of nice pants. Jeans are okay, but you're trying to impress, not lounge around and drink beer and eat peanuts. Women like men who know how to dress. Almost any color of shirt goes with khakis or dark casual pants—just stay away from loud patterns and stripes. Keep it simple. Don't complicate your life anymore than you have to.

As for shoes, buy a nice pair of leather dress shoes. Not the kind you wear with a suit but casual enough to wear with a pair of jeans or khakis. No French Shriners or Rockports either. If you're not sure of what kind of shoes to buy, just ask someone who works at a shoe store. Tell them what you're wearing them with (khakis, dark cotton casual pants etc.) If the sales person is a girl, she'll be more than happy to tell you what you need. You should also get some matching socks. A good rule of thumb is to match your socks to your shoes. And while you're at it, get a belt to match. Nothing looks worse than a guy wearing a brown belt with black shoes. If you don't get a belt that matches your shoes, you'll just look like any other jerk who doesn't know how to dress himself.

You can also get an idea of how to dress by observing stylish men. Go to any mall or night club or wherever and look for the guys who look like they have it together style-wise. These men, more than likely, will have a hot looking woman on their arms. In fact, she was probably the one who picked out his clothes. Learn from watching this guy. He's got a hot woman, doesn't he? He must know something you don't.

That's pretty much it when it comes to looking your best. Dress like this and you'll stand head and shoulders over a large percentage of the other guys who will be frequenting the establishments you're planning on going to. Most men don't know how to dress and the fact that you will be nicely dressed will make you stand out. If the girl you're talking to smiles and says something along the line of *"Who dressed you?"* take it as a compliment. She's saying that you actually look good, unlike the rest of dudes there.

In a nutshell, to dress nicely you will need:
- Nice shirt—keep it neutral—nothing loud or tacky.
- Nice pants—khaki's preferably.
- Good leather shoes.
- Matching socks.
- Matching belt.

Once you get your appearance straight, you'll need to work on your grooming and how you act around easy women. We'll discuss these aspects in the next couple of chapters. You just need to keep in mind that the emphasis on appearance is huge. You've heard how people say that women *like* men because they're funny. This may be true, but they have sex with men who look good and act like they care about their appearance. Keep in mind that if you don't care, she won't care either. That is, she won't care to bother talking to you, let alone have sex with you.

The best guy in the room: Hygiene and grooming.

If you're going to be the type of guy who gets laid a lot, you're going to have to look like the kind of guy who gets laid a lot. As, I've mentioned before, presentation is everything. This doesn't only include the clothes you wear but also your grooming and hygiene.

The main rule of hygiene is to be clean. Always be sure to shower and shave before you meet a potential casual sex partner. If you don't, you'll be the subject of one of her *bad date* stories. And when I say shower, I mean really clean yourself. Many men fall victim of the quick in-and-out when it comes to showering. They neglect to wash thoroughly. The main parts of your body to make sure you clean (and go back and clean them if you're in doubt) are your neck, underarms, ass, crotch and feet. Clean these and you'll most likely remove any potential odor. It goes without saying that you should always use soap and a washcloth. Also, don't forget the deodorant.

As with your clothing, when it comes to grooming, you should stay classic. I suggest that you always go clean-shaven and keep your hair short. Sure, some women prefer the long-haired, mustached rockstar look, but these women are in the minority. You'll attract more women by looking clean-cut. (I know you long-haired guys are going to hate this, but trust me. Ask any woman. Most men do not know how to care properly for long hair and it shows. It usually ends up looking greasy, unclean and unmanageable. And no, a ponytail holder does not fix these problems.) The main reason why women prefer clean-cut looking men is because they simply look cleaner and less threatening. It's a natural human reaction. This is why defendants always cut their hair before they go to court. Remember, looking for casual sex is just like going on a job interview. If you look like an axe-murderer, chances are you're not going to get an opportunity to speak to a woman. You need to make a good impression immediately. Don't question this dynamic. Just go with it and you'll be a much more successful person.

It's also not a good idea to pluck your eyebrows. Most men look absolutely ridiculous when they shape their eyebrows. Remember no woman wants a man who's trying to look prettier than she is. It is advisable however, if necessary, to get rid of your unibrow and trim any stray, crazy hairs that may grow wild from your eyebrows, ears, nose etc. Just don't shape them. This will only make you look silly and like you're trying too hard.

When it comes to cologne, I suggest that you should either keep it a minimum or avoid it completely. Many men think they must bathe in it, or least smell like they do. This is a quick way to get ridiculed by the opposite sex. Keep it to a minimum. You don't want your lady to suffer an allergic reaction when she takes a whiff of you, do you?

If you have a lot of tattoos, it's advisable to use common sense as to whether you highlight them or not. Many women love them, but if you're in more of a formal situation, it might be a good idea to keep them under wraps. Later, when you're getting more intimate, this can be a great topic of conversation. The old *I'll show you yours if you show me yours* routine. Women like showing off their tattoos as much as men do so this can be a great way to find common ground. Of course, the hope is that she'll get more than enough opportunity to look at them close-up. But if you're not sure, keep them covered until you are.

When it comes to earrings on men, I would say to take it out when you're on the prowl. It's not that I have anything personally against them, but some women don't really like them on men. Remember, you're trying to cast a wide net. If you find out that the girl you're after likes earrings, show her your hole and tell her that you're thinking about growing it in. That'll give her an opportunity to give her opinion and you the opportunity to get to know her a little better.

When it comes to grooming and hygiene, just remember to be classic and be clean. Most women aren't looking for a guy who looks like he stepped out of a sci-fi movie or off a rock and roll stage. They're looking for clean-cut guys who look like they want to have a good time. They don't want an oddball that they're going to have to figure out. Women are putting themselves at risk when they have sex with strangers so the more you look like a guy she can trust, the more likely you'll get laid. If you look like a serial killer, she's going to avoid you like the plague. Look like a guy, not like some guy who's trying to be something else.

The best guy in the room: Your physical appearance.

Getting laid is all about the physical. It's about that initial animal attraction. It's about you looking at a girl and, more importantly, her looking at you and knowing that yes, indeed, this is someone she wants to have sex with.

But if she doesn't do this when she looks at you, what happens?

You don't get laid, of course.

While we've discussed your clothes and your hygiene, there's one more aspect of your appearance that needs to be addressed. That's your actual physical appearance. You will have to look your best physically if you want to increase your chances of getting laid.

I know that everyone nowadays says that a person should accept themselves and not worry so much about exercising and losing weight. They say that it's okay to just be who you are and that people should love you for what you are inside rather than the way you look. This may be true in some cases, but if you want to get laid, you're going to have to get over these notions.

Sex is about the physical and the better you look physically, the more chances you will have of getting laid. If you're overweight, lose weight. If you're skinny, work out. It's that simple. Women are not turned on by couch potatoes. They like muscles. This is something you will have to accept. If you want to get laid, you will have to start working out. If you already work out, keep working out. I'm not going to go into any specific workout routines here because that's not the purpose of this book. I'm just telling you that if you want to get physical with a woman, you're going to have to start working on your physical appearance. If you're in doubt about what to do, join a gym and ask an expert. These people will be more than happy to help you get started.

The great thing about working out and losing weight is that once you get in the habit and start seeing some success, you will gain momentum and confidence. This will do wonders for your self-esteem which in turn will do wonders for your sex life. Also, you need to realize that working out will improve your ability to satisfy her. Easy women want strong men.

Another great thing about starting a workout routine is that it will help propel you into being the best man in the room. Most of the other guys who're trying to get laid will not be on any sort of exercise routine. They will be doughy, clueless and think that all they have to do is show up. You will definitely be at an advantage because it will be obvious to the females that you care about your body. If this isn't motivation enough for you, then what is?

If you're serious about getting laid, you also need to be serious about working out. Your physical appearance doesn't end with your clothes and hygiene. It also includes your body. The more in shape you are, the more sex you will have. It's that simple. Just be sure to consult with your doctor before embarking upon any new exercise routine.

Great places to find easy women: Hotel bars.

It's true.

Hotel bars are one of the best places to meet women on the prowl. Maybe it's the anonymity that a hotel affords two strangers or just simple convenience, but if you're looking to hook up, a hotel bar is a good bet.

The best kind of hotel bar to look for easy women is one near a convention center—or one that hosts a lot of business travelers. Usually women who are at conventions are of the same mind as the men who go to conventions. They're away from home and ready to party. The same thing goes with women business travelers. They get bored, they're alone and usually are up for a little something to take their minds off the tedium that is business travel. Hotel bars are also a good place to meet *Hotwives*. (See the chapter, *Easy women and some of their characteristics* for details.) These types of establishments offer a lot of opportunities for anonymous sex for these types of women.

Now of course, some of these women are going to be married, but that's not your problem. You're just there to make sure that they have a good time. One of the drawbacks to hotel bars is that, most likely, there are going to be a lot more guys than there are women. This is where your self-improvement comes into play. You have to be better than the pack. It won't take much effort, believe me. But you will have to put forth the effort if you want to be the biggest stud in the room.

So next time you're in a hotel, check out the bar. If you see a lady sitting by herself, send a drink over. Chances are she'll be more than happy to chat. After that, offer her another drink. If she accepts, you'll get a pretty good idea of whether she wants to party or not.

Don't aim too high.

I know this is something you probably don't want to hear but when you're looking for casual sex, you may have aim a little lower than you would if you were looking for a romantic long-term relationship. In other words, if you want to get some on a regular basis, you may have to lower your expectations.

But all the other how-to-get-laid books tell you how to pick up beautiful women and have sex with them without any effort, right? I hate to break it to you but most of the how-to-get-laid books out there are just pulling your leg. Unless you're absolutely rich or a male model or a rock star, it's going to be difficult for the average guy (in other words, *you*) to pick up a supermodel for a one-night-stand. Remember, there's no secret pick-up line or whammy you can put on her to change her standards. Besides, when it comes to casual sex, you don't want a girl like that. She's too high-maintenance and usually girls like that aren't even good lays. They don't have to be. They know all they need to do is show up and look pretty. They can also be quite bitchy and make you feel bad about yourself. You want the girls who are willing to work for your attention.

That's where aiming a little lower will greatly improve your sex life. Go for the girls who are interested in you. That's right. When you're going out on the town, pay attention to the girls who are actually conversing with you.

Sometimes they will be beautiful. Sometimes they will not. Regardless, if you want to get laid, you have to go with what you're attracting on any particular night. It's just like fishing. You never know what you're going to pull up until you actually go out there and reel one in.

There's a saying in the car business that goes: *"Always fuck your friends and family because you'll never get a chance to fuck your enemies."* The same thing goes with your interactions with women. You'll never get the opportunity to have sex with the women who don't want you. However, you'll stand an extremely good chance with the ones who do. And these women, most of the time, will be much better lays than the girls who think they're the most beautiful things in the world. They will put out and they will enjoy the attention you give them. So what if she's a little heavy or she wears glasses? Go for the personality. That's the true indicator of how good she will be in bed. If she's a cold fish in her conversation, then chances she'll be cold fish in bed. However, if she's a firecracker in her interactions, chances are she'll be hot in the boudoir. I've got a great example of this. One of the best strippers I've ever seen was a heavy-set Latina chick. She could work it like none of the skinny girls could. You could tell she really enjoyed being on stage and being sexual. As a result of this, you could overlook the fact that she had a few more pounds on her than the other girls. You want a woman who enjoys life and if a girl is starving herself to death or saving herself to be a trophy wife, she's not worth your effort.

All this is just common sense, but so many men out there just fail to follow it. The great thing about going for women in your league—or a little below it, even—is that the more women you pick up, the greater your confidence will grow. This alone will start getting you a better class of women. Just like it takes money to make money, it takes getting laid to get laid even more.

Heed this advice and lower your expectations and you will get laid. You may not have the Playmate of your dreams, but would you otherwise? Isn't getting laid better than not getting laid? Keep this in mind when you're out and about and thinking about snubbing the girls who you think are not quite up to your level. Get a reality check and realize that if she's interested in you and there's nothing obviously wrong with her, she's fair game. You'll probably have a lot more fun than you would with Miss America. She won't put out the way the girl-next-door will.

Internet options. The easiest way to get laid?

The internet has certainly made things easier, hasn't it? From ordering books to viewing porn, it's revolutionized the way we do everything. One area that's been especially improved because of the internet is that of *dating*—more specifically *dating for the purpose of casual sex.*

The internet abounds with ways to hook up. There are websites galore dedicated to casual sex and if you can't get laid via the internet, then you might want to take a look at yourself and what you're doing wrong. Maybe you need to improve or focus your approach or maybe you need to make some improvements in yourself. Regardless, with a few minor adjustments, you can get laid via the internet in no time. You just have to know how.

One of the greatest boons to casual sex that the internet has offered is in the fact that it has greatly desensitized us to the idea of sex though the omnipresence of porn and internet dating sites. It's just not that big of a deal for today's generation to have sex with no intention of establishing any other kind of relationship. What's especially great about this phenomenon is that it's not slowing down. I predict pretty soon, casual sex sites will go even more mainstream. It's happened with porn, hasn't it? It's just a matter of time before everyone gets in on the act.

Yes, there's definitely a new sexual revolution going on. It's almost like the sixties all over again. But what good is all this internet casual sex going to do you if you don't know how to get started? Well, there's no time like the present to get going.

What you need to do first is develop your profile. With this you need to be as honest as possible without getting too detailed. Be general in your information. Put in stuff like height, weight, etc. Just be sure to play up the good stuff, like your job (if it's a good one) or your athletic interests (if you have them). Just play up whatever hobbies or career you have to make them sound as interesting as possible. If you're an engineer, make what you're doing simple and exciting. Don't go into technical details that will only bore her. However, be sure not to say anything about your baseball card or *Disney* memorabilia collection. You want to avoid anything that will lead a woman to think you're anything less than a cool guy. You'll also have to get a good picture taken. It needs to be current. If it's one of you twenty years ago, you're wasting your time and hers. You need to keep it simple. Just one of you smiling and looking your best. Don't take one of yourself doing anything stupid or trying to be funny. It may not be interpreted as such. In the picture you want to accentuate your assets. If you have a good chest, wear a tight shirt. If you have a good smile, cheese for the camera. This is your first impression and how you'll sell yourself. If you don't have a good current picture, your chances of getting laid will wither. Remember these women are horny, not desperate. There are thousands of other guys out there just like you awaiting their shot. You have to put yourself at the front of the pack.

Next, you need to find an appropriate online dating site. This is probably the most crucial part of your internet dating adventure. You have to look specifically look for websites that cater to *Adult Dating* or casual sex. If you're not sure of where to find these sorts of sites, check out swinger's sites. They'll have links to these kinds of dating sites. Casual sex dating sites are the life's blood of swinging so you'll be able to get good information there. The biggest reason why you need to be careful with which site you choose is obvious. If you go with one of the mainstream dating sites, you're most likely going to be dealing with women who're looking for serious relationships. Sure, there might be some sex involved—eventually. But it'll most likely only occur after a lot of wining and dining. So pay attention. If you're after sex, go for the sex.

Of course, the next step is to place your ad. This much is self-explanatory.

After this, you'll have to figure out what exactly you're looking for. The biggest tip I can give you on this is to try not to be too picky or specific in what you want. If you are too specific, you'll eliminate some of the easy women out there unnecessarily. These are women who, if you saw them, you would definitely want to lay, but because you weren't looking for their type, they bypassed your ad. Remember what you're there for. Wait until she sends you a pic before you rule anyone out.

The next step is contact. Let's say that you search and find someone in whom you're interested. (It's a good idea to look for local women or at least women within driving distance for you, but hey, if you like to travel, go for it.) You want to send her a message. The important thing here is to not come off as sounding weird, creepy or perverted. Be a gentleman. Tell her about yourself and that you're interested in meeting her. If she replies that she's interested, send a pic. As a man, you'll most likely have to send the first pic. This is just the way it is, so get used to it. If things spark and you're both interested, set up a meeting. Unless she specifically asks you to choose the place, let her. Typically most women are much more comfortable picking the setting. After that, the rest is up to you. It should be no secret what you're both interested in. Remember, this why you chose an *adult* dating site. Just try to make a good impression. Be smooth, buy her drink, pay for her food and be nice. And don't be too aggressive. Make no assumptions that she is automatically going to have sex with you. Never allude to the fact that that's all you're there for. It's a good idea to let her lead in this regard. She'll let you know if she's interested. It won't take a lot of effort for this girl to put out. This is what she's here for. Just don't give her a chance to turn you down

One thing to understand is that if, for whatever reason, a woman doesn't respond to your photo favorably or possibly doesn't even respond to your email at all. don't worry about it or take it personally. You're probably just not her type. There are plenty more women out there. Move on to the next one. You don't want to waste your time on the ones that aren't interested in you, anyway.

Of course, you will have to keep in mind, as in most cases of casual sex, there will far more men on the internet seeking casual sex than there will be women. This is why you have to be patient and you have to work on yourself so you stand out. Dress well and be polite and you will make yourself much more desirable and likely to get laid than you would have otherwise.

All you have to remember when it comes to casual sex is that if you've got a computer and can be honest, the world is truly your oyster. All you have to do is sell yourself and put your best foot forward. Internet dating is like a singles bar that's always open. All you have to do is play your cards right and you'll be hitting it in no time.

Chivalry is not dead. The way to keep getting laid.

As I keep saying, if you want to get laid, you've got to stand out from the pack. You have to be that guy that is above the rest. Because, let's face it, most women can get laid whenever they want. But us guys have to work at it. After you've made yourself into the guy who the easy girl wants to lay, how do you get her to keep letting you come back for more?

It's easy. Be a gentleman.

You heard me right. Be a gentleman. Remember, it's all about her. You're just along for the ride, so to speak. Do a good job and satisfy her properly. Let her orgasm before you. Buy her drinks and food. Open her door and let her talk. All these things are key to you being perceived a gentleman. When you're a gentleman, there's little chance of you becoming anyone's bad memory. Keep in mind that it's all about having fun and creating those good memories. Treat her nice and you will be guaranteed to become one of her booty calls. And she will become one of yours. She may even become a friend. An actual friend with benefits.

That's what you're shooting for. You want to develop that network of girls with whom you can have casual sex and you will do this if you can be a nice guy. Yes, you heard me. You will have to be a nice guy. No, I'm not talking about the nice guy that people push around. I'm talking about the nice guy who's a considerate casual sex partner.

As you work your way through this book and develop yourself into a *casual-sex-getting-laid* kind of guy, your confidence and ability will grow. You will acquire the traits that women look for in a casual sex partner. Sure, some women love jerks, but you're not looking for that kind of relationship. Remember, this is just about sex. Not about anything romantic. The girl has to trust you and if you're a gentleman, she will.

So, when you're with a girl, just keep in mind to be nice and considerate. This way, she'll be more than happy to invite you back for more. It's just like networking in the business world. The more contacts and favorable impressions you make, the more likely you are to get laid.

How to know if she's ready.

So, you're in the right place at the right time. You're surrounded by easy women who are just aching to have sex. The only problem is how do you know if they want to have sex with you? How can you tell if you're the guy for them? How can you tell if you're clicking?

In other words, how can you tell if she's *ready*?

Since this is an important step before you make your move, it's a good idea to get your bearings straight before you try to seal the deal. Luckily for you, she'll most likely let you know that she's ready. She'll probably pull you aside and flat out tell you. This is especially true considering that most of these girls like to feel that they're the ones in charge. And also, it gives some of them a kick to make the first move.

However, if she's a little bit old-fashioned, you'll just have to look for some subtle signs. These will be most likely expressed by her body language. She'll flick her hair or make a lot of eye contact. She may start to mirror your actions—like looking at her watch after you look at yours, lighting a cigarette after she sees you light one, etc. Also, she may touch your arm or other body part. Believe me, it happens. Please bear in mind that these are just some of the basic indicators of attraction. If you want more in-depth information regarding body language, consult a book or website dedicated to the subject.

If she's truly old-fashioned, she might also just give you her phone number. If you have a good feeling that she'll be more willing to go a bit farther in a different setting, go for it.

It'll be different for different women, so try not to get too nailed down to specific gestures. Just follow your instincts and if you think she's ready, try to seal the deal. And if you're wrong, it's no problem. At least you won't be wasting your time on someone who isn't going to be putting out.

How to seal the deal.
Moving from the bar to the bedroom.

Okay, you've done everything right and she's really vibing on you. You know she's interested but what do you do next? How do you get her back to the boudoir? (Or at least to an empty stall in the ladies room?)

Most of the time, with a loose woman, this isn't going to be an issue. She'll let you know what she wants and will lead you into the situation. Most easy women are very proud of the power they hold over men and relish every opportunity to show it. However, if she's playing a little hard to get, it could be that she isn't sure whether you're ready to party or not. When this happens, you'll need to work yourself into a situation where you're both on the same page and ready to have sex.

While the situations will be different, what'll you need to do will essentially be the same regardless of the scenario. You'll have to get her into a slightly more intimate setting for the two of you to let nature happen. Of course, this approach doesn't apply to any trysts you're having on camera with an internet amateur or encounters with prostitutes, but I'm sure you already figured that out. What I'm talking about here is what needs to happen when you meet a woman in a bar, a swing club or on an internet date.

The main thing to remember is that if you are to get laid, you will need a pair of balls. That is to say, you will need the guts to start to the ball rolling in the direction you want the situation to go. If the two of you are clicking, that is if she's *ready*, there are several options for you to do this. If you're in a place where there's dancing, ask the girl to slow dance. This will be a great opportunity for the two of you to be close and will allow her to let her hands do the walking. If there's no dancing, just try to find a secluded place in a bar. When she's out of the way of prying eyes, she'll be much more likely to show you how she really feels. If neither of these options work, take a walk in the park or anywhere else where there's not a lot of people. Of course, she'll have to be interested in you or she won't go anywhere alone with you, so be careful. More than likely, the situation will not be so ambiguous. You'll know which way the wind's blowing. Remember, don't push. If she doesn't want to go anywhere with you, just say that it was nice to meet her and move on. You don't want to waste your time on a situation that's not going to work out.

Of course, if you're lucky, you won't have to go through any of these preliminary steps and she'll invite you up to her place straight from wherever you met her. Or she may even suggest that the two of you get a room. (You should always pay if this is the case. Remember what I said about being a gentleman?) Most easy women just want to cut to the chase. If not, just read the situation and play it by ear. No one can tell you step by step how to get laid, but you can listen to the advice of those who know and greatly increase your chances.

But what if you get her up to her place and are at a loss as to what to do? Whether you're a virgin or just inexperienced, what if you're at loss as how to proceed? I don't think you should worry about this because she'll lead the way. Just go with the flow and do what comes naturally. Also, I personally recommend you pick up a book on sexual technique and watch some instructional films—porn, in other words. The main thing is to exercise some self-restraint. Remember you're not at an all-you-can-eat buffet. Make sure that your partner gets satisfied and the rest will take care of itself. If you orgasm early, just make sure that she has an orgasm too. You can do this by oral or manual stimulation. Apologize for orgasming too quickly by saying that she just turned you on too much. You wouldn't be lying, would you?

So, when it comes to sealing the deal, just use your instincts. Chances are that there will be no doubt that the girl wants to have sex with you, but if there is, just try to get her into a more private setting. Once she feels safe from the judgmental eyes (unless she's an attention seeker, of course) of the public, she'll be more than happy to invite you up.

No means no. How to handle rejection.

How do you feel whenever someone asks you to do something you don't want to do? You decline because you don't want to do it, but you're polite about it, right? Now, think about this for a second. How do you feel when they ask you again? And again? And again? How about when they start threatening you? You don't like that very much and you don't want to have anything more to do with this person, do you?

Well, this is something to keep in mind when you're out on the prowl. If you're chatting up some chick and she turns you down, just let it go. If you keep bugging her, you'll only make yourself look bad. Plus, you'll spoil your reputation with her friends and everyone will think you're a jerk.

Some guys out there get so frustrated that they'll even start threatening a woman. They think just because they bought her a drink that she owes them something. They get hung up and think, *"I have to have this woman! She has to let me sleep with her!"* In other words, they start acting like psychos. Well, if you're one of these guys, you need to get your head straightened out. A guy like this is not going to get laid very often and most likely will end up in jail. You don't want to viewed like this, do you? Never threaten a woman. It's a low-class thing to do plus it's completely counter-productive to getting laid. Besides, you don't want everyone to think you're a creep do you?

And then, on the other hand, there are the desperate guys. They beg and they whine when they're turned down. *"C'mon, just give me a chance,"* they'll say. Don't be this guy. This never works. The idea of the mercy fuck is one that mostly exists in the fantasies of the incompetent. No woman wants to get laid by a desperate loser when there are confident guys who lined up around the corner. If you ever feel the impulse to grovel, slap yourself and get out of there. If you embarrass yourself like this, it will be almost impossible to recover.

Everyone gets shot down. Regardless of how easy the woman is, there are going to be some who just won't warm to you. Maybe it's the color of your hair or that you remind her of someone else. This is something you're just going to have to accept as part of the game. Whenever it happens, just be a gentleman and smile and act like you don't care. Be cool. Bear in mind that while this one didn't want you, there are plenty out there who will—that is if you don't make an ass out of yourself with the ones who don't. The wonderful thing about it is, is that if you're confident enough and a gentleman about it, this chick might just change her mind— or she might introduce you to her friends. Remember what you're there for. You're there for the sex. You don't want to burn any bridges.

The moral of the story is that when she turns you down, don't try to put on the hard sell. Don't act desperate and don't grovel. Just play it off and act cool. Never let the façade of confidence drop. You're not selling vacuum cleaners, you're selling yourself. And when you're selling yourself, desperation, belligerence and lack of self-awareness are never good selling points. Don't ever threaten. Remember she can always call the cops. A night in jail is never a good way to end an evening. Just be confident, shake off the rejection and move on to the next one. If you keep up this approach, those doors will eventually open for you.

Great places to find easy women: The Club.

You know the scenario. You are out on the prowl. It's Friday night and you've got your paycheck burning a hole in your pocket. You want to have a good time and meet some women. So where do you go? Why, the club, of course.

It's pretty obvious that if you want to meet people who want to party, you go to *where* they party. It's just common sense. And of course, where there are people partying, there are women who are looking to get laid. There's alcohol and dancing and everything else that turns women on. But is going to a night club a sure thing? No, not on your life.

One of the biggest problems with using the club (AKA the Meat Market) to find easy women is also one of its biggest drawing points—the opportunity to meet lots of women. Why this is a problem is that many of the women you'll meet will not be easy. They will not be there to get laid. They will be looking for serious long-term relationships. They will be there with friends. They will be there with people they work with. There are any number of reasons why these women will be at a night club. And chances are some of these women will be easy enough to lay after a little bit of partying, but to get them you're going to have to meet quite a few that aren't.

When going to a night club to party, always keep in mind that you need to meet as many women as possible. You don't need to get hung up on just talking to one—unless, you hit the jackpot right off the bat. The longer you spend talking to one girl, the less your chances are of meeting easy women. They will see you as taken and not available. You don't want this. Talking to just one girl is good if you're looking for a relationship, but if you're looking to get your rocks off, you need to be out there mingling. You need to put yourself out there as the guy who likes to party. However, there's one thing to keep in mind when you're mingling, don't be too obvious that you're looking for sex. If you are, the girls will catch on to you pretty quickly and the night will be over for you. Just be smooth and be friendly. And discreet. Remember, you're just having fun and meeting people. This is why you're mingling. If you take this approach, you'll meet a lot more people. The girls who are interested in you will let you know.

To find these easy women, you need to use the skills you'll learn in this book on how to seal the deal and how to know when they're ready. It'll be pretty obvious which girls are there to party and which ones are there just to tease. Remember, if a girl rejects your advances, don't worry about it. Be a gentleman and move on to the next one.

While the club is a great place to meet women, just realize that not all women there will be easy. Use your instincts and keep your mind focused on the task at hand—getting laid. If you do this, you'll be able to wade through all the girls who are there just to waste your time.

The much celebrated, but greatly overrated wingman.

I know. I know. You always need a buddy. You need that guy to handle the not-as-attractive friend while you're going for the hot chick. Well, while it's good to have a friend in on the action, it's not always necessary when it comes to casual sex. In fact, sometimes it can even hurt your chances of getting laid.

The concept of the *wingman* is usually applied to the normal meeting in a bar for the purpose of a regular relationship-type encounters. Sure, in these types of scenarios, you might end up having sex, but usually it's just drinking and having a good time while the girl and her pals evaluate you and your wingman. You might go out later, but then again, maybe not.

However, in a strictly casual sex scenario, your friend might just scare off the girl. She might think that you and your friend are evaluating her or the other girls at the club. She might even think you're gay. When you go to a swing club or a bar/meat market alone, you're much more likely to meet women than you are otherwise. When you go alone, you're forced to interact. Whereas, with a friend, you can always retreat into the little world of baseball scores and *Star Wars* talk that you two share. However, if you're alone and confident to talk to women and buy them drinks, you'll probably get invited over to a table. But this will not work unless you make the effort to talk to people. You have to use that confidence to buy drinks and start up conversations. These people are here to meet people too. Otherwise they would have just stayed at home. Just start talking to the ladies a few times and you'll see what I mean. Once you start going to these places alone and start mingling, you'll soon find out that your wingman was probably nothing but dead weight.

While friends are nice, you need to get out of that pack mentality when it comes to casual sex. In this type of situation, a wingman will just hurt your cause. He may even take it upon himself to intervene and take the girl for himself. This is definitely not a good situation for you. Remember, you're not there to get him laid. You're there to get laid yourself. When you look at it from this perspective, the wingman just isn't worth the trouble. Just think about it this way: You don't need someone to hold your hand when you go to the bathroom, do you? Neither should you when you're trying to get laid.

Friends with benefits?

As human beings we all want friends, but as horny men we especially want friends with benefits. You know, female friends that with whom we can have sex.

Okay, in case you've been under a rock for the last few years, a *friend with benefits* is a friend of the opposite sex who will have sex with you. No strings attached. In previous years it was called the *booty call* among other things. The reality of it is that while we have heard of people having friends with benefits—mainly from the television—rarely do we actually know anyone who actually has one of these. I personally have known only a few people who have been able to attain such companions and I know a lot of sleazy individuals.

I almost put this chapter in the ones with the myths about getting laid, but it's not really a myth. It is actually something that can happen. However, it's just not that common or something you can count on. Like anything else, it depends on the company you keep and if you're not keeping company with easy women (which I'm assuming you're not since you're reading this book), most likely, you're not going to have one of these.

But let's say that, for example, you do develop a friend with benefits. What then? Well, I say take advantage of it while you can and tread lightly. Chances are, if your friend with benefits is indeed a friend, she's going to want to be more than just a friend after she dishes out the benefits a few times. Many times a girl, for whatever reason, will have sex with a guy she's interested in under the guise of just two friends *getting together*. I think the main reason for this is because she wants the guy but she doesn't want to scare him off. She knows that very few men are going to turn down sex so there you have it. If you want a relationship with your friend with benefits, then you're in luck. If not, you may find yourself in a sticky situation and will probably lose the friendship unless the two of you are mature enough to work through things.

And on the other hand, if you're having sex with your friend, you might be the one who starts becoming attached. Friends usually do have a common affection for one another and this is the primary basis for a relationship. This is understandable, but if she doesn't care for you in this way, you might just end up with your feelings hurt. You might want to think twice about going in this direction unless you've got a good feeling that she might feel the same way.

So, friends with benefits? Maybe, but usually the benefits will ultimately have strings attached. Go into it with both eyes open and don't be surprised if she or you want to take things further than the friend stage. Just be prepared because, when you involve sex in your friendships, things can get a little more complicated than you might like.

Girls' night out? I don't think so.

The girls' night out.

It's the stuff of dreams, isn't it? You and your buddies are out on the town and you go to a club and find a group of girls out getting drunk and having a good time. You would think when a bunch of girls are out going wild that it would be easy pickings for a guy on the make such as yourself.

Think again.

Chances are if you run upon a gaggle of girls when you're out and about, you're not going to stand a chance in hell of getting laid. I know it runs contrary to what you might think because you're thinking of them the same way you and your buddies think of yourselves when you're out. All you're thinking about is partying and getting some. Girls aren't like this. Unless you hit the jackpot of a group of easy women, most likely, the only action you're going to be getting is when they accept your drink and then make fun of you for sending it over. They're not going act the slut when they're all together because, unlike you, they have reputations.

Now, it's possible that you might be able to exchange numbers with one of these girls, but most likely, it's only because she's interested in you as someone that she could potentially have a serious relationship with. If this is okay with you, great. Just don't be shocked if she's refuses to be your booty call.

Of course, if you run upon a group of easy women out partying, all your dreams will come true. But, of course, this is the kind of thing that usually happens only in the confines of porno films. While this is something in the realm of possibility, chances are it's not going to happen in real life.

So the rule of thumb is not to expect much when you happen upon a girls' night out. They're most likely not interested in having a good time with anyone other than themselves. Even if they are complete sluts they aren't going to act like it around their friends. No one likes to be talked about like that.

Do you wanna be in pictures? Another way to get laid courtesy of the internet.

If you're interested in sex, chances are you look at porn on the internet. And if you look at porn on the internet, chances are you've seen the websites of internet amateurs. And if you've looked at any of the sites for any period of time, you'll note that many of them have will have sex with selected members of their sites. And also with anyone who is willing to show his face on their sites. If you're willing to let yourself be photographed on camera, this is a good way to have sex.

If you're not sure what internet amateurs are, they're usually ordinary women who have websites featuring them doing sexual things. These sites run the gamut from women simply taking their clothes off to them having sex with lots of men and women. Many times these women are also swingers. This is the type of woman who will be more likely to have sex with you.

The way you get chosen to be on an internet amateur's site is quite simple. You apply. Many webmistresses have actual applications on their sites. Usually they will state what they're looking for. If you fit the bill, go for it. Other sites will not have anything like this. For these sites, it's best to write a thoughtful, well-composed business-like email stating your purpose and that you're willing to be shown on her site doing sexual things with her. Of course, you should not expect to be compensated in any way monetarily. You're getting to have sex. That's your payment. There's no way that she's going to pay you for having sex with her. Just understand this up front before you make a fool of yourself by asking. If she's interested, she'll reply back. Don't send a pic unless/until she asks for one.

Many of these internet amateurs are married or in serious relationships, so there is a sleazy element involved. However, many of them are quite hot so this should help you overcome the sleaze factor. If she replies to you, the best approach to being one of the guys she chooses to have sex with for her site is to be a gentleman. (I know I keep saying this, but it's that important). Don't be pushy or say lewd things to her. Use the same qualities you would when you're trying to get laid by anyone else. This will greatly improve your chances. Just let her and her husband/boyfriend call the shots. Remember, they're just gathering content for the site while you're getting laid. This is something to keep in perspective.

If you choose to go this route, don't be surprised if you're not treated that well by either the husband or the internet amateur. To them, you may just be a piece of meat. Just someone to exploit on the internet. If you can handle this aspect of it, you'll be okay. Just don't take it personally. At least you're getting some, right?

There are many ways to get laid via the internet and being a stunt cock (always wear a condom!) on an internet amateur's website is just one of the many. If you can handle the sleaze and having your pic out there for millions to see, it can be a good way to go. And just think, if you do a good job, she'll probably tell her other internet amateur friends about you. This could lead up to you getting laid a lot.

Dirty tricks.

Regardless of the setting, whether it's the club, a party or wherever, there are certain things you can say to easy women to reveal just how easy they are. These kinds of things could almost be considered dirty tricks. Due to the fact that I think that they are sort of underhanded, I don't necessarily recommend them. However, I thought it best to include them just in case you feel the need to manipulate a woman into some sort of lewd act for your pleasure. But, on the other hand, you're probably not getting her to do something that's she's not already done a bunch of times with a bunch of other men. So maybe they're aren't really that devious after all. Regardless, you should beware when you use these little tricks. They will work so be careful of the woman you use them on. You never know when a girl is a psycho, a stalker or has a jealous boyfriend/husband.

When resorting to the dirty tricks, two major factors need to be in play. The woman has to be easy and she has to be somewhat interested in you. You'll get the first one sorted by being in the right place and observing the signs that indicate a woman's level of sluttiness. (See the chapter on *Easy women and some of their characteristics.*) And you'll get the second one covered by following my tips on improving yourself. After you get these under control, the ball is in your court.

Now about the particulars of the dirty tricks. These are simple statements that play upon certain young women's insecurities and inability to overcome peer pressure. They will prey upon the desire of the young women to be a *bad girl* and to shake off her old self-perception as a goody-goody-two-shoes.

I'm just going to include a few of these to give you an idea of what they entail. You can vary them or create new ones in the same vein. But as I mentioned earlier, be forewarned. If you say these around easy women who you're aren't really interested in, you might find yourself in a situation that you hadn't counted on.

Here's a few phrases that can manipulate an easy woman into having sex with you:

"I'm impotent." Tell this to some slutty women and they'll be sure to prove that you aren't. She'll show that you may not be able to get it up with most girls, but *she* won't have a problem in that area.

"I'm celibate." This one works similar to the "*I'm impotent*" phrase except that easy women will do their damnedest to get you to break your vow of chastity.

"I'm a virgin." This one works the same as the previous one. An easy woman who's somewhat interested in you will be more than willing to be your *first*.

"You seem like such an innocent, sweet girl." If you say this around a girl who is insecure and obviously *not* an innocent, sweet girl, you will probably at least get a hand job out of the deal. This plays on the fact that some women, for some reason, want to be *bad*.

"I'm saving myself for marriage." All slutty women can't wait to deflower a man and show him that sex isn't that big of a deal. They look at it as an educational experience. You should look at it as your good fortune.

Now, of course, you can't just blurt these phrases out nonsensically. You have to work them into your conversation. If you don't, you'll just come off as sounding socially awkward and inappropriate. Be smooth. You'll get your opportunity. Especially if the girl's interested in you.

When it comes to these dirty trick phrases, just keep in mind that you can't say them around all women and receive the response you're looking for. If you say them around a bona fide good girl, she'll probably empathize with you and thank you for saying that she's a good girl. However, if you use them around a genuinely loose woman who's mildly interested in you, it might unlock a Pandora's Box like you wouldn't believe. But she has to be interested because if she isn't, she won't give a damn either way about your impotence. As I mentioned earlier, I don't really believe in manipulation, but you have to look at it this way: These women are going to have sex with somebody so why can't it be you? And if you can say something that speeds along the process, it shouldn't be something to lose sleep over.

Great places to find easy women: Nudist resorts.

While nude beaches are not considered to be very good places to get laid, nudist resorts are a different story entirely. Of course, this is not to say that they're a sure thing, but going to one can definitely increase your chances of casual sex.

The thing to realize is that many nudists are also swingers. And if they're not swingers, they're at least fairly open-minded. And while many nudist resorts are family affairs where mom and dad can bring the kids, they're also places where people can relax and let it all hang out. And I'm not just talking about shuffleboard, either.

Because of the family atmosphere of many of the nudist resorts, most of the freaky stuff happens late at night after all the youngsters are in bed. Now, of course, there are some nudist resorts where there is absolutely no funny business allowed, but if you do a little research on the internet (I suggest nudist, naturist and swinger message boards as good resources) you will find the ones where this kind of crazy stuff happens. This will be word-of-mouth information because no resort will actually advertise that wild sex occurs after hours. I personally would recommend that you steer clear of family-oriented places, because they're more likely to be uptight. But this is just my opinion and I can't speak for all of them.

The main difference when it comes to the getting laid factor between nude beaches and nudist resorts is that going to a nudist resort requires a higher level of commitment than most single guys are willing to make. This weeds out a lot of the *tourists* and shows that you indeed are willing to participate.

Since many of the people who will be interested in casual sex at a nudist resort are swingers, keep in mind that the same rules apply as with swing clubs. No means no and don't be pushy. Remember that some swingers don't like single guys so always show proper respect to the couples. Nudists are typically very social. Just be a cool guy and you're bound to start interacting with the people there. I do not recommend that you bring up any talk of casual sex or swinging to anyone at a nudist resort because there's always a possibility that this kind of talk can get you kicked out. What I would recommend is just going to where the people are partying. This can be happening at the pool, the clubhouse or someone's room. Regardless, the important thing is to keep in mind that there will *always* be a place where people are partying and you just need to find it. If there's anything happening it will be where people are drinking and having a good time. And I definitely recommend going to the party places late at night.

Once of the big drawbacks of nudist resorts are that many of the people there are older. This isn't to say that everyone is, but you will see a large number of people in their fifties and sixties. I don't know why this is, but it's just the way it is. But don't let this discourage you because there will also usually be younger people there as well. Just accept that older people are especially attracted to nudism and you won't be surprised.

One thing you need to realize is that there is a possibility that if you go to a nudist resort, you will not even get the opportunity to talk about casual sex. If not, don't sweat it. At least you got to see the show and get a little sun. The best way to approach going to a nudist resort is to not go looking for sex, but for the experience. Just be sure to go to where the partying is and if there's something going on, you'll know that you're poised to join in.

Let the big head do the thinking. The dangers of the easy lay.

Have you ever heard the phrase that if something's too good to be true, it usually is? While it's not true all the time, it can definitely apply to casual sex.

What a bringdown, you think.

But it's true. If you don't go into casual sex with both eyes open, you can set yourself up for a lifetime of regret. The little head doesn't always think very clearly when it's presented with a beautiful opportunity to get laid without any effort. This is why you have to let the big head take over.

So what are the pitfalls?

You should always be aware when you're picking up a girl for casual sex that she's not a prostitute. Legitimate prostitutes will tell you up front. But there are some who are unscrupulous who won't let you in on what's going on until after the fact. If you don't have a problem with her being a working girl, more power to you. At least she's a guaranteed lay. However, if she lets you do your thing and starts demanding money after the fact, so to speak, she's probably just shaking you down. I would recommend trying to get the hell away from her. But if you can't without her shooting or stabbing you or calling the cops or her pimp, pay up and chalk it up to inexperience. You'll know better next time.

Another danger of the easy lay is that she might be a con artist. Especially if you're the type of guy who doesn't necessarily want to be known as the casual sex type. I'm not going to pass judgment here, but if you're a politician, minister, teacher etc., you really might want to think twice about doing the casual sex thing. If you want to fool around, go somewhere where absolutely no one knows you and hire a prostitute. And don't tell anyone or try to write it off on your taxes. If you're in a sensitive professional situation and you do insist on a life of easy lays, just be aware that a girl who is a little too eager could be working to blackmail you. I know that this is not necessarily the most sexy thing to think about when you're looking to get your rocks off, but if you've got something to lose in getting laid, you need to be very careful where and with whom you do it.

Another danger is that of the scorned wife/girlfriend with issues. If you run upon a girl who's dying to have sex with you, she might just be trying to make someone jealous. This someone might be a homicidal ex-husband or boyfriend. Be careful and don't get too attached. It's hard to avoid this one, but just try to look for clues like if she says that her previous boyfriend was jealous or if she says that he used to be in prison. Just be careful and if you have any suspicions, maybe don't go back around her for a while just to see if you're right.

One of the most celebrated, but unlikely dangers of the easy lay is the kidney/organ thief. While is it is a little farfetched, it has happened. Everyone has heard of the story of the guy meeting a knockdown gorgeous girl in a bar and going back to her place only to blackout and wake up in a bathtub with a hole in his body where his kidney used to be. This is a hard one to watch out for because it's so rare and unlikely. The key thing is to just watch what you drink. Especially if you're in a strange place or a strange country. A good rule of thumb is to never leave your drink unattended regardless of the setting. Don't worry unnecessarily though because if she drugs you, she'll probably just steal your wallet. But you don't want to take any chances.

There are many other scenarios when an easy lay might come with a price, but while the details may be different, the gist of them isn't. Just be aware of the company you're keeping. If a girl is overly friendly or too eager, something funny might be up. Just pay attention and trust your instincts. If something doesn't feel right, it probably isn't. Whether the girl is a con artist, has issues or is an organ thief or just a bad time, go into casual sex with your eyes open. Try to stay sober and if you think something is up, run for it. Listen to your gut instinct. It's usually right.

Great places to find easy women: Science fiction conventions.

Science fiction? Getting laid? Surely, I'm out of my mind.

It would seem that way. Common sense tells you that there's nothing quite so mutually exclusive than science fiction and the act of getting laid, but the fact of the matter is that there are quite a few loose women at science fiction conventions. Many of these girls are eggheads who were quite the goody-goodies growing up and now that they're adults, they're out to let the world know that they are ready to party. Also the fact that they're probably either atheists or Wiccans doesn't hurt your chances too much either.

Typically science fiction conventions attract not only people who are interested in science fiction, but also fans of fantasy role-playing, medieval weaponry/life, comic books, witchcraft and many other fringe subjects. These sorts of interests are very attractive to many loose women. And even if some of them are complete dorks, many of them won't be. Many of them will think nothing of having sex with complete strangers if it fits into the lifestyle they envision for themselves.

Also, there's usually a lot of alcohol being consumed at these things, so that ups the getting laid probability quite a bit. Many people also have *room parties* in the hotels where these conventions are held, so most likely it will be quite a festive atmosphere. Always research a convention on the internet before you go to get an idea of what to expect. Some conventions are not necessarily known for their parties, so be aware of this before you go. You don't want to waste your time on the wrong kind of convention.

Another good thing about science fiction conventions (aside from the fact that this is the one place it is okay to talk about your *Star Wars* fixation) is that most of the guys there are going to be complete dweebs so it's very easy to be one of the best guys in the room. This fact alone will be one of your greatest assets.

As with any great place to get laid, just go in for the experience and don't go in looking for sex. Try to go where the people are partying and if there are easy women around, they'll most likely find you. If they don't, just enjoy the freak show.

Bad boys versus nice guys.

It's the truth. Women seem to love men who treat them badly. This is not only true of women who are looking for relationships but also women who are looking for sex. They just love the bad boy. They love the guy who looks like he's more likely to steal more than just her heart.

So how's a nice guy like you supposed to get laid?

First of all, you have to understand that women only *seem* to love men who treat them badly. Lots of nice guys get laid all the time. This is because they know how to act and present themselves with confidence and authority. You've heard of the *Knight in Shining Armor*? He's certainly not a jerk. The reason why many women go off with the bad boy instead of the nice guy is because given a choice between the two, the bad boy seems much more likely to be a better lay. The truth hurts, but this is the way it is. A lot of nice guys just don't have the confidence to approach women in the right manner. They come off as wimps or as ineffectual. Women hate wimps. They also hate dorks. You have to remember that when they're looking for a sexual partner, they're working on a primitive level. Back in the caveman days, having an encyclopedic knowledge of New York Yankees World Series trivia just wouldn't have been enough to persuade her to come back to your cave.

"*But I've tried! The asshole always gets the girl!*" I know that you're saying this as you read these words, but you need to know that he's not getting her because he's an asshole.

He's getting her because he's more confident and presents himself better than you. It's tough to hear this, but you need to know before you move on. Once you get over your hurt feelings and try a little self-examination, you'll see that your luck will start turning around. You can always improve yourself. If you're failing at picking up women, something is wrong and chances are it's in how you present yourself. Everyone can make improvements. You just have to get over your ego and realize that it's not an admission of defeat to make yourself better. It's an adjustment that will work to get you laid.

So what are you to do? You're not a Neanderthal, right? A leopard can't change its spots. Yes, this is true, but you can clean up your act. Dress more fashionably (consult your men's magazines for ideas) study movies starring cool guys and go on a field trip to a bar and try to observe how the bad boys operate. Be chivalrous. Actually be a *Knight in Shining Armor*. Buy her drink. Open her door. Light her cigarette. And always do it with confidence. Do it with an air of, *"I know how to treat a woman, unlike the rest of these jerks. That's because I'm a man, not a naughty little boy."* It's fairly simple. Most women, given the choice between a bad boy and confident, nice guy, will pick the nice guy every time.

Set your goal on being the *Knight in Shining Armor* rather than the doormat and you'll see that nice guys do indeed get the girl. It may take some work on your part, but do a little self-study and try to figure out where you're going wrong. Getting laid and picking up women is just like anything else. You have to work at it. You have to hone your skills and practice. Build up your confidence and reinvent yourself as a confident guy. Nice guys do get laid. Wimps and dorks don't. It's that simple. Change how people perceive you and you'll greatly increase your odds in the bedroom.

Spring break?

Anyone can get laid at spring break. We've all seen the exploitation movies so we know it has to be true, right?

While this isn't necessarily always the case, it can be sometimes. This is why I'm including it in this book.

The reason why spring break can be a great place to get laid is due to the party atmosphere, the large amount of alcohol involved and the fact that so many people are coming together who will probably never see each other again in their lives. Anonymity and alcohol usually lead to sex whenever the opposite sexes are involved.

It's that simple. If you're a nice-looking guy who has taken care of his body and has worked on making himself the *best guy in the room*, you will have a good chance of getting laid. All it takes is a little confidence and you should be in. The only caveat is that you will have to be around college age for this to work. A middle-aged guy cannot and should not attempt to go to spring break and attempt to get laid. He will just look pathetic and will probably draw much undue attention to himself. Sometimes, if he goes too far, he might find himself being attacked by some of the younger people. He may even be perceived as a pervert and this is never good.

So, if you're young enough, spring break is a good bet at getting laid. But if you're past that point, just go on vacation at some other time. You never want to come across as being pathetic. Pathetic never gets you laid.

Prostitutes.

If you're absolutely desperate and you feel completely incompetent around women (and you've have no experience at all with women and are absolutely intimidated by the thought of being with a woman), you can always call in a professional.

Yeah, you heard me correctly. You can go to a prostitute.

A prostitute is a guaranteed way of getting laid and it can do wonders to help clarify the mystery that is *woman*. I think that if you're a man who's of a certain age who hasn't had the good fortune to be with a woman, it is advisable to go to a working girl. She is a professional and can help you get up to speed.

Of course, like with anything, there are a few things you need to know about prostitutes. I would stay away from street hookers or even unauthorized escort services. These are illegal and many of the girls are not necessarily motivated by ethics of hard work and a retail economy, if you know what I mean. These types of prostitutes may possibly rip you off, rob you or, even worse, give you a disease. If you're going to hire a prostitute, go to a first world place where it is legal, like Nevada or Amsterdam or other various places in the world. You can research legitimate brothels and etiquette on the internet. These girls are tested and have to do business in a professional way. Also, they are in it for the money and they will make sure you are satisfied. Otherwise, it adversely affects their professional reputation. It's a business for them and the customer has to be taken care of. If you're going to spend a lot of money on getting laid, you want to make sure that it's worth every penny.

As with all women, always treat the prostitute you hire with respect. She is a lady and even though some narrow-minded men have a tendency to look down on them, just remember that she is providing a service that you are buying. Without someone like you there would not be someone like her. These women have families and are normal people at heart, so do not be mean or condescending. Be nice and it'll only enhance your experience.

But one thing to remember is that you don't want to start relying on prostitutes as the sole way to satisfy your sexual needs. This will break you financially. Also, do not ever fall in love with one. This is just a business to her. Do not be under any illusions that you are going to rescue her from her horrible life. You will only get hurt and cause her a lot of problems. Besides this a very condescending way of looking at things. Have fun, but keep it a professional relationship and just think of the sex as a service she's providing. You just want to do this to get back in the game. After you do this, take the principles you learn in this book and from your newly reaffirmed confidence and go out there and do it for yourself. Pick up your own one-night stand. Hiring a prostitute is not the end. It is only the beginning of casual sex for you.

So in a nutshell, if things aren't working out for you and you don't know which end is up (literally), go to a legal professional sex-worker. A prostitute is a good way to demystify sex and to let you know that it is not that big of a deal. Remember to be a good guy about it and always thank her for a good time. Never start solely relying on prostitutes as your source of sexual fulfillment. This can get quite expensive. Know when to say when and get yourself back out in the real world.

The Mercy Fuck. A myth that will not get you laid.

If you're like me, you were probably brought up on raunchy teen comedies where nerds perform some sort of mojo and the chicks just fall into bed with them. It's just that easy. Well, as you've probably figured it out, getting laid does not happen like it does in these teen sex farces. While it's not that difficult, it does require a little finesse. However, as long as you continue to believe in some of these myths of getting laid, you'll never be able to come into your own.

You have to realize at the heart of these myths of getting laid is the notion that you can just fall into a casual sex situation without having to have any sort of redeeming qualities or making any sort of effort. This is ridiculous. Sure, when you start out in your casual sex lifestyle, you will happen upon situations where you will seem to just fall into sex. But you have to realize that this will not happen all the time and when it does, you're falling into them because you've laid the proper groundwork. You've made yourself into a better person. You've made sure you're in the right place to find easy women and you've developed your confidence. It's very easy to confuse this effort with luck.

When it comes to myths, there is none greater than that of the Mercy Fuck. You gasp, "*Say it ain't so.*" Well, it is. It's simply not true. The idea that a girl will have sex with you simply because she feels sorry for you is not really based in reality. I'm not saying it hasn't happened, because it probably has. But then again, somebody wins the lottery every now and again too. Get the point?

Look at it this way: A girl feels sorry for you and thinks you're so pathetic that the only way you'll ever get laid is for her to just lay down and let you do her. Do you realize how preposterous this is? A girl doesn't want to have sex with a guy she feels sorry for when there's some other confident guy around who she figures can really give her what she's looking for. Women have no problem getting laid. They're not like us. All they have to do is put it out there and we're all over it. Since this is the case (and you know it is) why would she go with somebody she doesn't respect or isn't interested in? You do the math.

There are a lot more myths out there that I won't go into, but I think you get the idea. Anytime you hear about some guy getting laid with no effort or no redeeming features is probably just a load of bull. If it's too good to be true, it probably is. Just keep this in mind and you'll stay much more focused in reality. And reality is the place where you're most likely to get laid.

But what if she wants a real relationship?

While most of the time it's the guy who falls in love, there will inevitably be exceptions to the rule. Even the easiest of women want to be loved. This is just an essential part of who we are as human beings. So, if you do happen to develop a *friend with benefits* or just a regular hook-up, it's bound to come up. She wants to have a *real relationship*. When this happens, what do you do?

This one is especially easy. Just do what you feel like doing. If you like the girl and think that you can make it work, go for it. If not, tell her that you're not ready for that step right now. But whatever you do, don't disrespect her and tell her that while she's the type of girl you like to have sex with, she's definitely not the type that you want to have as a girlfriend. Remember to be a gentleman at all times. Even when you're the one who's doing the rejecting.

But if you're even the slightest bit interested, think long and hard before you reject her. She just might be the type of girl that's just right for you—loose, easy and crazy about sex. There's a lot of virtue to those vices. Just think about how she complements your lifestyle. You never know when the girl you're having random sex with might just be the one.

What we've learned.

At this point in the book, I think it's important that you should review what we've discussed. This is a brief overview of what you should know when you're embarking on a life of casual sex. It is merely a list of the main topics and is not meant to be complete, but rather the key points that we've covered.

Key points:
- You're not a eunuch, don't act like one. It's okay to want sex.
- Get your priorities straight. Understand just exactly what are you looking for in a relationship.
- Understand what you will need to know in order to get laid.
- Picking up women is not a magical process. It can be learned by anyone.
- Know the types of easy women. They usually fall into one category or another.
- Easy women are to be respected and revered. They are still ladies. They just like sex and aren't afraid to go after it.
- Always wear a condom. You don't know where a girl has been.
- Health screenings are good. Make sure that you get them regularly.

- If you want to have a lifestyle of casual sex, you will have to overcome the Sleaze Factor.
- There will be more men than women interested in casual sex. This is why it's important for you to stand out.
- If you want to get laid, you have to hang out with sluts. Easy women are much likely to have sex with you than uptight ones. Go for the loose ones.
- If you want to pick up loose women, you'll have to go where the loose women are. There are some places where you're more likely to get laid. These are the places with high concentrations of loose women.
- Understand that there are places where you *will not* stand a chance of getting laid regardless of what you've seen in porno movies and on TV.
- You will have to develop confidence in order to get laid.
- How you present yourself is crucial in whether you get laid or not.
- You have to know how to approach an easy woman.
- Don't use pick-up lines. They're too risky—and cheesy.
- Develop your script. In other words, have an idea of what to say when you approach a woman.
- Keep yourself in check around women with whom you want to have sex. Don't come on too strong or too desperate.
- Understand that, in order to be the best man in the room, you will have to work on improving your wardrobe, your hygiene and your physical appearance.

- The internet is a great way to meet women for casual sex whether it's through adult dating or through having sex with internet amateurs.
- Don't set your expectations or standards too high. You want women who are accessible to you and are pleased that you're interested in them. Women who don't like you most likely will not have sex with you.
- Remember to always be a gentleman.
- You have to know when a woman is ready for your advances. If you don't, you'll get shot down rather swiftly.
- Know that there is a system to sealing the deal.
- Wingmen are overrated and largely unnecessary.
- Learn how to handle rejection.
- Friends with benefits are great, but sometimes there are strings attached.
- A girls' night out is not usually a good thing for a guy who wants to get laid.
- Some dirty tricks will help you get laid. But be careful who you use them on.
- It's a good idea to stay sober when you're on the prowl. You don't want to do anything that you might have avoided if you hadn't been drunk.
- Sometimes there's more to the easy lay than first appears. Be aware of the dangers that casual sex can entail.
- A confident nice guy will always get the girl over the bad boy.
- Prostitutes are a great way to get oriented into a lifestyle of casual sex. Just realize that they are just a means to get back in the saddle. Don't rely on them to fulfill your sexual needs.
- The mercy fuck is largely a myth.

- Understand that any sexual relationship can lead to a real relationship. This can either be a good or bad thing for you depending on what you want. Be ready for this situation to develop.

Please refer back to the body of the book for further explanations and a more complete coverage of each key topic.

In conclusion.

So now you know how to get laid. It wasn't that big of a mystery after all, was it? Most people find that after they get laid a few times, it just isn't that big of a deal for them anymore. I mean, they still want to do it, but they aren't quite so mystified by the process. And that's exactly what the purpose of this book is: To cut through all the crap and show men how they can pick up easy women.

Most of the time, the reason why men can't get laid is because of they've listened to bad advice or watched too many teen exploitation movies. Real life isn't like that. While it is quite unpredictable at times, most of the time you can move within its uncertainties to operate towards your goal. It's not that difficult once you get you start making an effort. All you need is a little bit of confidence and a basic knowledge of easy women and you're in. You also have to bear in mind that if you want to get laid, you have to go to where the easy women are, but you've got this down pat, right? I hope so.

Now that you're no longer in the dark, you should be able to look at those clueless fools at the night club with nothing but pity. You'll be content in the knowledge that you're now in the know and no longer out there chasing your tail. But since you're on your way to *Casual-Sex-ville*, this leads to the question, *"Where do you go from here"?* Do you become a regular horn dog on the prowl? Or do you bide your time until the right easy chick comes along? It's up to you. The world is indeed your oyster and if you paid attention while you were reading this book, you should be ready to open it.

You're not a eunuch. It's okay for you to want to get laid. Just keep in mind that while casual sex is a lot of fun, it can also be dangerous if you don't take precautions. Also, be respectful of others and know when to back off. Just because one woman doesn't want you, doesn't mean that there isn't another that's just dying to have you come on to her.

Good luck and stay safe.

Printed in the United States
103837LV00001B/196/A